Philip McCallion, PhD, ACSW
Editor

Housing for the Elderly: Policy and Practice Issues

Housing for the Elderly: Policy and Practice Issues has been co-published simultaneously as *Journal of Gerontological Social Work*, Volume 49, Numbers 1/2 and 3 2007.

Pre-publication
REVIEWS,
COMMENTARIES,
EVALUATIONS . . .

"**V**ery important . . . carries the message that getting it right has very serious implications for public policy and for the individual. . . . They also provide us with important ways to think about this individual and ethereal notion of quality of life."

Neal E. Lane
Former Director of the New York State Office for the Aging and a partner with Optimum Partners Consulting

More Pre-publication
REVIEWS, COMMENTARIES, EVALUATIONS . . .

"**M**AKES AN IMPORTANT CONTRIBUTION to ongoing federal and state discussions, offering unique perspectives on how the Olmstead ruling's potential for fairness and integration can be applied to older Americans. The empirically-based discussions of NORCs and assisted living programs add new levels of data and texture to ongoing program design issues and related policy debates, as well."

James F. O'Sullivan
Sr. Program Officer, John A. Hartford Foundation, New York

The Haworth Press, Inc.

Housing for the Elderly: Policy and Practice Issues

Housing for the Elderly: Policy and Practice Issues has been co-published simultaneously as *Journal of Gerontological Social Work*, Volume 49, Numbers 1/2 and 3 2007.

Monographic Separates from the *Journal of Gerontological Social Work®*

For additional information on these and other Haworth Press titles, including descriptions, tables of contents, reviews, and prices, use the QuickSearch catalog at http://www.HaworthPress.com.

Housing for the Elderly: Policy and Practice Issues, edited by Philip McCallion, PhD, ACSW (Vol. 49, No. 1/2 and 3, 2007). *A comprehensive look at how housing is changing to support the growing number of elderly persons in the United States.*

Elder Abuse and Mistreatment: Policy, Practice and Research, edited by M. Joanna Mellor, DSW, and Patricia Brownell, PhD (Vol. 46, No. 3/4, 2006). *"IMPORTANT. . . . Rarely does a single book offer the reader the wealth of information and the multidimensional perspective of this collection. The contributors are academicians and practitioners in the variety of fields whose involvement is now understood to be vital to an effective response to a growing problem. Their contributions provide practical tools to professionals in several disciplines, and put forward concrete methodologies for screening, assessment, and intervention." (Betty F. Malks, MSW, CSW, Director, Santa Clara County Department of Aging and Adult Services, San Jose, California; North American Regional Representative, International Network for the Prevention of Elder Abuse)*

Religion, Spirituality, and Aging: A Social Work Perspective, edited by Harry R. Moody, PhD (Vol. 45, No. 1/2 and 3, 2005). *"From the definitive opening chapter by the eminent social gerontologist David Moberg to the erudite final chapter by Eugene Bianchi, the breadth and depth of this collection of essays provide a major contribution to the understanding of religion, spirituality, aging, and social work. These essays will both inform and challenge the reader." (Dr. Melvin A. Kimble, PhD, Professor Emeritus of Pastoral Theology and Director, Center for Aging, Religion, and Spirituality, Luther Seminary, St. Paul, Minnesota; Editor of Viktor* Frankl's Contribution to Spirituality and Aging)

Group Work and Aging: Issues in Practice, Research, and Education, edited by Robert Salmon, DSW, and Roberta Graziano, DSW (Vol. 44, No. 1/2, 2004). *Although there is a considerable amount of writing on both group work and social work with the elderly, there is surprisingly little about applying this practice method to this specific age group.* Group Work and Aging: Issues in Practice, Research, and Education *fills this gap by presenting penetrating articles about a mutual aid approach to working with diverse groups of older adults with varied needs. Respected experts and gifted researchers provide case studies, practice examples, and explanation of theory to illustrate this practice method with aging adults, their families, and their caregivers. Each well-referenced chapter delivers high quality, up-to-date social group work practice strategies to prepare practitioners for the needs of the growing population of elderly in the near future.*

Gerontological Social Work in Small Towns and Rural Communities, edited by Sandra S. Butler, PhD, and Lenard W. Kaye, DSW (Vol. 41, No. 1/2 and 3/4, 2003). *Provides a range of intervention and community skills aimed precisely at the needs of rural elders.*

Older People and Their Caregivers Across the Spectrum of Care, edited by Judith L. Howe, PhD (Vol. 40, No. 1/2, 2002). *Focuses on numerous issues relating to caregiving and social work assessment for improving quality of life for the elderly.*

Advancing Gerontological Social Work Education, edited by M. Joanna Mellor, DSW, and Joann Ivry, PhD (Vol. 39, No. 1/2, 2002). *Examines the current status of geriatric/gerontological education; offers models for curriculum development within the classroom and the practice arena.*

Gerontological Social Work Practice: Issues, Challenges, and Potential, edited by Enid Opal Cox, DSW, Elizabeth S. Kelchner, MSW, ACSW, and Rosemary Chapin, PhD, MSW (Vol. 36, No. 3/4, 2001). *This book gives you an essential overview of the role, status, and potential of gerontological social work in aging societies around the world. Drawing on the expertise of leaders in the field, it identifies key policy and practice issues and suggests directions for the future. Here you'll find important perspectives on home health care, mental health, elder abuse, older workers' issues, and death and dying, as well as an examination of the policy and practice issues of utmost concern to social workers dealing with the elderly.*

Social Work Practice with the Asian American Elderly, edited by Namkee G. Choi, PhD (Vol. 36, No. 1/2, 2001). *"Encompasses the richness of diversity among Asian Americans by including articles on Vietnamese, Japanese, Chinese, Taiwanese, Asian Indian, and Korean Americans." (Nancy R. Hooyman, PhD, MSW, Professor and Dean Emeritus, University of Washington School of Social Work, Seattle)*

Grandparents as Carers of Children with Disabilities: Facing the Challenges, edited by Philip McCallion, PhD, ACSW, and Matthew Janicki, PhD (Vol. 33, No. 3, 2000). *Here is the first comprehensive consideration of the unique needs and experiences of grandparents caring for children with developmental disabilities. The vital information found here will assist practitioners, administrators, and policymakers to include the needs of this special population in the planning and delivery of services, and it will help grandparents in this situation to better care for themselves as well as for the children in their charge.*

Latino Elders and the Twenty-First Century: Issues and Challenges for Culturally Competent Research and Practice, edited by Melvin Delgado, PhD (Vol. 30, No. 1/2, 1998). *Explores the challenges that gerontological social work will encounter as it attempts to meet the needs of the growing number of Latino elders utilizing culturally competent principles.*

Dignity and Old Age, edited by Rose Dobrof, DSW, and Harry R. Moody, PhD (Vol. 29, No. 2/3, 1998). *"Challenges us to uphold the right to age with dignity, which is embedded in the heart and soul of every man and woman." (H. James Towey, President, Commission on Aging with Dignity, Tallahassee, FL)*

Intergenerational Approaches in Aging: Implications for Education, Policy and Practice, edited by Kevin Brabazon, MPA, and Robert Disch, MA (Vol. 28, No. 1/2/3, 1997). *"Provides a wealth of concrete examples of areas in which intergenerational perspectives and knowledge are needed." (Robert C. Atchley, PhD, Director, Scribbs Gerontology Center, Miami University)*

Social Work Response to the White House Conference on Aging: From Issues to Actions, edited by Constance Corley Saltz, PhD, LCSW (Vol. 27, No. 3, 1997). *"Provides a framework for the discussion of issues relevant to social work values and practice, including productive aging, quality of life, the psychological needs of older persons, and family issues." (Jordan I. Kosberg, PhD, Professor and PhD Program Coordinator, School of Social Work, Florida International University, North Miami, FL)*

Special Aging Populations and Systems Linkages, edited by M. Joanna Mellor, DSW (Vol. 25, No. 1/2, 1996). *"An invaluable tool for anyone working with older persons with special needs." (Irene Gutheil, DSW, Associate Professor, Graduate School of Social Service, Fordham University)*

New Developments in Home Care Services for the Elderly: Innovations in Policy, Program, and Practice, edited by Lenard W. Kaye, DSW (Vol. 24, No. 3/4, 1995). *"An excellent compilation. . . . Especially pertinent to the functions of administrators, supervisors, and case managers in home care. . . . Highly recommended for every home care agency and a must for administrators and middle managers." (Geriatric Nursing Book Review)*

Geriatric Social Work Education, edited by M. Joanna Mellor, DSW, and Renee Solomon, DSW (Vol. 18, No. 3/4, 1992). *"Serves as a foundation upon which educators and fieldwork instructors can build courses that incorporate more aging content." (SciTech Book News)*

Vision and Aging: Issues in Social Work Practice, edited by Nancy D. Weber, MSW (Vol. 17, No. 3/4, 1992). *"For those involved in vision rehabilitation programs, the book provides practical information and should stimulate readers to revise their present programs of care." (Journal of Vision Rehabilitation)*

Health Care of the Aged: Needs, Policies, and Services, edited by Abraham Monk, PhD (Vol. 15, No. 3/4, 1990). *"The chapters reflect firsthand experience and are competent and informative. Readers . . . will find the book rewarding and useful. The text is timely, appropriate, and well-presented." (Health & Social Work)*

Twenty-Five Years of the Life Review: Theoretical and Practical Considerations, edited by Robert Disch, MA (Vol. 12, No. 3/4, 1989). *This practical and thought-provoking book examines the history and concept of the life review.*

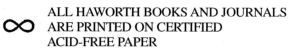

Housing for the Elderly: Policy and Practice Issues

Philip McCallion, PhD, ACSW
Editor

Housing for the Elderly: Policy and Practice Issues has been co-published simultaneously as *Journal of Gerontological Social Work*, Volume 49, Numbers 1/2 and 3 2007.

The Haworth Press, Inc.

www.HaworthPress.com

Housing for the Elderly: Policy and Practice Issues has been co-published simultaneously as *Journal of Gerontological Social Work,*® Volume 49, Numbers 1/2 and 3 2007.

The development, preparation, and publication of this work has been undertaken with great care. However, the publisher, employees, editors, and agents of The Haworth Press and all imprints of The Haworth Press, Inc., including The Haworth Medical Press® and Pharmaceutical Products Press®, are not responsible for any errors contained herein or for consequences that may ensue from use of materials or information contained in this work. Opinions expressed by the author(s) are not necessarily those of The Haworth Press, Inc. With regard to case studies, identities and circumstances of individuals discussed herein have been changed to protect confidentiality. Any resemblance to actual persons, living or dead, is entirely coincidental.

The Haworth Press is committed to the dissemination of ideas and information according to the highest standards of intellectual freedom and the free exchange of ideas. Statements made and opinions expressed in this publication do not necessarily reflect the views of the Publisher, Directors, management, or staff of The Haworth Press, Inc., or an endorsement by them.

Library of Congress Catalog-in-Publication Data

Housing for the Elderly: Policy and Practice Issues/ Philip McCallion, editor.
    p. cm.
"Housing for the Elderly: Policy and Practice Issues has been co-published simultaneously as Journal of gerontological social work, Volume 49, numbers 1/2 and 3 2007."
Includes bibliographical references and index.
ISBN 13: 978-0-7890-3448-9 (hard cover : alk. paper)
ISBN 13: 978-0-7890-3449-6 (soft cover : alk. paper)
    1. Older people--Housing–United States. 2. Older people--Services for -- United States. 3. Older people–Housing–Canada. 4. Older people–Services for–Canada. I. McCallion, Philip.
HD7287.92.U54H686 2007
363.5′9460973–dc22
                                         2007024299

The HAWORTH PRESS Inc

Abstracting, Indexing & Outward Linking

PRINT *and* ELECTRONIC BOOKS & JOURNALS

This section provides you with a list of major indexing & abstracting services and other tools for bibliographic access. That is to say, each service began covering this periodical during the the year noted in the right column. Most Websites which are listed below have indicated that they will either post, disseminate, compile, archive, cite or alert their own Website users with research-based content from this work. (This list is as current as the copyright date of this publication.)

Abstracting, Website/Indexing Coverage . . . . Year When Coverage Began

- *(IBR) International Bibliography of Book Reviews on the Humanities and Social Sciences (Thomson) <http://www.saur.de>* **2006**

- *(IBZ) International Bibliography of Periodical Literature on the Humanities and Social Sciences (Thomson) <http://www.saur.de>* **1996**

- ***Academic Search Premier (EBSCO)** <http://search.ebscohost.com>* **1993**

- ***Applied Social Sciences Index & Abstracts (ASSIA) (ProQuest CSA)** <http://www.csa.com>* **1987**

- ***CINAHL (Cumulative Index to Nursing & Allied Health Literature) (EBSCO)** <http://www.cinahl.com>* **1981**

- ***CINAHL Plus (EBSCO)** <http://search.ebscohost.com>* **2006**

- ***Expanded Academic ASAP (Thomson Gale)*** **2001**

- ***Expanded Academic ASAP - International (Thomson Gale)*** . . . **1989**

- ***Expanded Academic Index (Thomson Gale)**.* **1992**

- ***InfoTrac Custom (Thomson Gale)*** **1996**

- ***InfoTrac OneFile (Thomson Gale)*** **1989**

- ***MEDLINE (National Library of Medicine)** <http://www.nlm.nih.gov>* **2005**

(continued)

(continued)

(continued)

(continued)

Bibliographic Access

- **Cabell's Directory of Publishing Opportunities in Psychology** *<http://www.cabells.com>*

- **Magazines for Libraries (Katz)**

- **MedBioWorld** *<http://www.medbioworld.com>*

- **MediaFinder** *<http://www.mediafinder.com/>*

- **Ulrich's Periodicals Directory: The Global Source for Periodicals Information Since 1932** *<http://www. bowkerlink.com>*

Special Bibliographic Notes related to special journal issues (separates) and indexing/abstracting:

- indexing/abstracting services in this list will also cover material in any "separate" that is co-published simultaneously with Haworth's special thematic journal issue or DocuSerial. Indexing/abstracting usually covers material at the article/chapter level.
- monographic co-editions are intended for either non-subscribers or libraries which intend to purchase a second copy for their circulating collections.
- monographic co-editions are reported to all jobbers/wholesalers/approval plans. The source journal is listed as the "series" to assist the prevention of duplicate purchasing in the same manner utilized for books-in-series.
- to facilitate user/access services all indexing/abstracting services are encouraged to utilize the co-indexing entry note indicated at the bottom of the first page of each article/chapter/contribution.
- this is intended to assist a library user of any reference tool (whether print, electronic, online, or CD-ROM) to locate the monographic version if the library has purchased this version but not a subscription to the source journal.
- individual articles/chapters in any Haworth publication are also available through the Haworth Document Delivery Service (HDDS).

As part of
Haworth's
continuing
commitment
to better serve
our library
patrons,
we are
proud to
be working
with the
following
electronic
services:

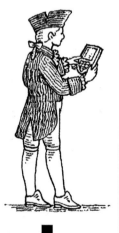

AGGREGATOR SERVICES

EBSCOhost

Ingenta

J-Gate

Minerva

OCLC FirstSearch

Oxmill

SwetsWise

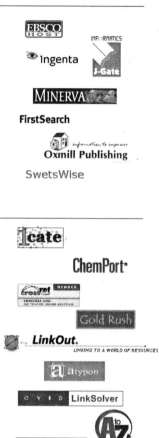

LINK RESOLVER SERVICES

1Cate (Openly Informatics)

ChemPort
(American Chemical Society)

CrossRef

Gold Rush (Coalliance)

LinkOut (PubMed)

LINKplus (Atypon)

LinkSolver (Ovid)

LinkSource with A-to-Z (EBSCO)

Resource Linker (Ulrich)

SerialsSolutions (ProQuest)

SFX (Ex Libris)

Sirsi Resolver (SirsiDynix)

Tour (TDnet)

Vlink (Extensity, formerly Geac)

WebBridge (Innovative Interfaces)

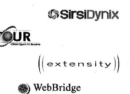

Housing for the Elderly: Policy and Practice Issues

CONTENTS

THE OLMSTEAD DECISION

*The Olmstead Decision of 1999 continues to have the potential to radically trans-
form the long-term care system in the United States. This article will review the
components of the decision and steps being taken by the federal and state governments to address its challenges and mandates. A number of key areas where social
workers can play important roles will be described.*

KEYWORDS. Olmstead decision, long-term care, disabilities, social work roles,
community integration

NATURALLY OCCURRING RETIREMENT COMMUNITIES

ABOUT THE EDITOR

Philip McCallion, PhD, ACSW, is Professor in the School of Social Welfare at the University at Albany, a Hartford Geriatric Social Work Faculty Scholar and Mentor and Director of the Center for Excellence in Aging Services. Dr. McCallion's research on aging is focused on the interaction of informal care with formal services, strategies for the maintenance of quality of life, and the experiences of multi-cultural families. Dr. McCallion's research has been supported by grants and awards from the National Institute on Drug Abuse, the John A. Hartford Foundation, the Agency for Health Quality and Research, the U.S. Administration on Aging, the Alzheimer's Association, The Joseph P. Kennedy Jr. Foundation, the Health Research Board of Ireland and New York State's Department of Health, Office for the Aging, Office for Children and Family Services and Developmental Disabilities Planning Council.

Dr. McCallion has published on interventions with caregivers of frail elderly, persons with Alzheimer's disease, and persons with developmental disabilities. He is co-editor of *Grandparents as carers of children with disabilities: Facing the challenges*, co-author of *Maintaining Communication with Persons with Dementia* and has produced videotape and cd-rom-based training and self-instructional materials on Intellectual Disabilities and Dementia. Dr. McCallion has also written on management issues for the providers of human services. He is co-editor of *Total Quality Management in the Social Services: Theory and Practice*.

Foreword

Joanna Mellor and I present this volume with absolute certainty that it will become must reading for all social work practitioners, administrators, academics, and researchers who are interested in and/or want to gain expertise in issues having to do with housing for older people. Our much valued colleague, Philip McCallion, has done an extraordinary job of editing this volume. He was able to interest/recruit/entice/bamboozle a group of true experts in housing to write chapters for the book, chapters which address practice and policy concerns from a variety of points of vantage, and his Preface is worthy of a careful read.

The Section on "The Olmstead Decision" contains three chapters which are particularly helpful, we believe, to social workers interested in understanding the impact of Olmstead, and each of the chapters in the other sections similarly will serve to stimulate the interest of our readers, and increase our understanding of policy and practice issues in this very important domain.

Dr. McCallion welcomes your comments about this volume, and Dr. Mellor and I congratulate him on the excellence of his work.

Rose Dobrof, DSW

Joanna Mellor, DSW

[Haworth co-indexing entry note]: "Foreword." Dobrof, Rose. Co-published simultaneously in *Journal of Gerontological Social Work* (The Haworth Press, Inc.) Vol. 49, No. 1/2, 2007, p. xxiii; and: *Housing for the Elderly: Policy and Practice Issues* (ed: Philip McCallion) The Haworth Press, Inc., 2007, p. xix. Single or multiple copies of this article are available for a fee from The Haworth Document Delivery Service [1-800-HAWORTH, 9:00 a.m. - 5:00 p.m. (EST). E-mail address: docdelivery@haworthpress.com].

Available online at http://jgsw.haworthpress.com
xix

Preface

It is increasingly regarded as a truism that the majority of aging persons would prefer to spend their later years where they have always lived. It is also true that for many seniors in the U.S. that they will move often for quality of life reasons to new types of housing and new locations as they age. The manuscripts contained here seek to capture some of the key aspects of the transitions aging persons experience and how housing programs may contribute to the maintenance of quality of life. In some areas the research the manuscripts summarize what is known, in others they are opening issues to research for the first time. A third group of papers captures form the perspective of social workers several key policy issues, particularly the unfolding impact of the Olmstead decision.

As we anticipate the first wave of Baby Boomers crossing the threshold of age 60, there is growing recognition of the realities of increasing percentages of individuals in many U.S. states living to older ages and of aging persons representing a growing proportion of many state populations. For society, this represents an important and valued outcome of improving health care and services, as well as of improved pension and health insurance schemes. The contributions of many individuals in choosing more healthy lifestyles should also be recognized. Indeed for many seniors, a long, productive, healthy and enjoyable old age is possible.

Just as the arrival at this state of affairs is the result of both societal and individual factors, the same forces will shape the types of lives experienced by seniors in their older years. The following manuscripts seek to capture this interaction of society and the individual as it pertains to housing and to offer some insight on the role social workers may play to ensure productive and enjoyable aging.

The manuscripts in Part I fall into three areas:

Setting a Housing Context. Alley and colleagues set a context for the other papers by discussing the increasing interest in aging or elder friendly/prepared communities and they report on a Delphi study identifying the most important characteristics of such communities. Setting a context would not be complete,

[Haworth co-indexing entry note]: "Preface." McCallion, Philip. Co-published simultaneously in *Journal of Gerontological Social Work* (The Haworth Press, Inc.) Vol. 49, No. 1/2, 2007, pp. xxv-xxvii; and: *Housing for the Elderly: Policy and Practice Issues* (ed: Philip McCallion) The Haworth Press, Inc., 2007, pp. xxi-xxiii. Single or multiple copies of this article are available for a fee from The Haworth Document Delivery Service [1-800-HAWORTH, 9:00 a.m. - 5:00 p.m. (EST). E-mail address: docdelivery@haworth press.com].

xxi

however, without highlighting forgotten and at risk populations. Here, McDonald and colleagues address homelessness issues among older people, Ramos links housing disparities and caregiving issues with the aging of older Puerto Ricans and Kolomer and Lynch report on the challenges experienced by grandparents who late in life become the primary caregivers of their grandchildren.

The Olmstead Decision. At a time when advocacy and social change through the courts is judged more limited than in early decades the Olmstead Decision stands out as an important potential mechanism for change for both people with disabilities and older persons. Three papers explore this decision and its implications for the living situations of older persons and for the advocacy roles of social workers. Palley and Rozario address how frail older persons may be included in the ADA definition of persons with disabilities and the Decision's implications for long term care. Zendell describes the current state of change and roles social workers may play. Finally, Yong places Olmstead in the context of a policy journey toward greater integration, discusses how social work has changed as a result and challenges social workers to continue to accordingly evolve practice.

Naturally Occurring Retirement Communities. The evolution of Naturally Occurring Retirement Communities (NORCs) has sufficiently advanced that it was possible to bring together three manuscripts that review what is known about this phenomenon. MacLaren and colleagues review the experience in New York State of developing and operating supportive service programs. Cohen and colleagues offer a typology and set of principles for the integration of services in housing, particularly low income housing. Finally, Carpenter and colleagues report on the re-location concerns of older adults living in a suburban NORC.

The manuscripts in Part II fall into two areas:

Housing Outcomes. Assisted living is a newer form of housing alternative for the elderly and one which is often not equally available to seniors resulting in advocacy for extension of this option to all. Zimmerman and colleagues report on their extensive investigation of whether assisted living facilities meet their goals of providing both privacy and support. Kelley-Gillespie and Farley also report on an exploratory study of the effect on perceptions of quality of life when individuals are moved from nursing home to assisted living facilities.

Historical Perspectives. The final manuscript provides an historical perspective on housing issues for the elderly. In reconnecting with the contributions of Harriet Tubman, Crewe reminds us of the double jeopardy historical discrimination represents for the housing of older African Americans.

The manuscripts taken together represent an overview of critical issues in housing for the elderly and will hopefully encourage future research, policy efforts and redesign of practice.

This introduction would not be complete without recognizing the efforts of Lisa Ferretti, MSW, from the Center for Excellence in Aging Services who managed the review and editing process and acknowledging the support to the guest editor offered by the John A. Hartford Foundation, the U.S. Administration on Aging, the New York State Department of Health and the New York State Office for the Aging.

Philip McCallion, PhD
Editor

Creating Elder-Friendly Communities: Preparations for an Aging Society

Dawn Alley, BS
Phoebe Liebig, PhD
Jon Pynoos, PhD
Tridib Banerjee, PhD
In Hee Choi, MA

SUMMARY. Because many communities where older people live were not designed for their needs, older residents may require support to remain in the least restrictive environment. "Age-prepared communities" utilize community planning and advocacy to foster aging in place. "Elder-friendly communities" are places that actively involve, value, and support older adults, both active and frail, with infrastructure and services that effectively accommodate their changing needs. This paper presents an

The authors are very grateful to Serena Sanker for her work on the Delphi study and to Gretchen Alkema and Christy Nishita for their insightful comments and suggestions. This work was supported by a grant from the Provost's Office of the University of Southern California.

[Haworth co-indexing entry note]: "Creating Elder-Friendly Communities: Preparations for an Aging Society." Alley, Dawn et al. Co-published simultaneously in *Journal of Gerontological Social Work* (The Haworth Press, Inc.) Vol. 49, No. 1/2, 2007, pp. 1-18; and: *Housing for the Elderly: Policy and Practice Issues* (ed: Philip McCallion) The Haworth Press, Inc., 2007, pp. 1-18. Single or multiple copies of this article are available for a fee from The Haworth Document Delivery Service [1-800-HAWORTH, 9:00 a.m. - 5:00 p.m. (EST). E-mail address: docdelivery@haworthpress.com].

Available online at http://jgsw.haworthpress.com
doi:10.1300/J083v49n01_01

1

analysis of the literature and results of a Delphi study identifying the most important characteristics of an elder-friendly community: accessible and affordable transportation, housing, health care, safety, and community involvement opportunities. We also highlight innovative programs and identify how social workers can be instrumental in developing elder-friendly communities. *doi:10.1300/J083v49n01_01 [Article copies available for a fee from The Haworth Document Delivery Service: 1-800-HAWORTH. E-mail address: <docdelivery@haworthpress.com> Website: <http://www. HaworthPress.com> © 2007 by The Haworth Press, Inc. All rights reserved.]*

KEYWORDS. Community assessment, neighborhood, aging services, planning, age-prepared

INTRODUCTION

In the next 20 years, more Americans will live into advanced age and the large Baby Boomer cohort will move into retirement. By the year 2020, about one in five Americans will be over age 65 (Kinsella & Velkoff, 2001). Some areas, including rural communities and retirement destinations, will include even larger concentrations of older persons. This explosive growth of older adults represents both opportunities and challenges at the community level.

An aging population presents an opportunity because many older adults are committed, long-time residents who contribute their time and energy to local issues. The majority of older adults are homeowners, and over 60 percent have lived in their homes for at least 11 years (Bayer & Harper, 2000). Approximately 86 percent of older adults give to charity organizations, over one-third participate as volunteers, and almost 20 percent provide informal care to a friend or family member (Feldman, Oberlink, Simantov, & Gursen, 2004). Communities can use planning to create an environment that supports and capitalizes on this "elderpower." If communities support aging in place through appropriate infrastructure, older adults can be empowered to continue as active citizens and volunteers for many years, enriching communities through their time and experience (e.g., delivering in-home meals to persons with disabilities, caring for grandchildren).

However, supporting aging in place may be a challenge for many communities. "Aging in place" refers to individuals growing old in their own homes, with an emphasis on using environmental modification to compensate for limitations and disabilities (Pynoos, 1993). Ideally, older adults should not have to move to be in a supportive environment. Over 80 percent of older adults express a desire to remain in their own homes as long as possible (AARP, 2000).

Yet, aging in the community may not be possible without community support, because older persons frequently experience declining capacity for independent living. In 1997, 27 percent of community-dwelling Medicare beneficiaries over 65 experienced difficulty performing one or more activities of daily living (e.g., walking, eating, toileting); more than half of Americans over 85 experience these limitations (U.S. Administration on Aging, 2003). Even more older adults experience difficulties with instrumental tasks such as driving and shopping. As physical or cognitive capacity declines with age, older persons may need additional support to maintain their independence. For citizens aging with a disability, the ability to carry out daily tasks and participate in community life is often dependent on accessible infrastructure and social resources.

Faced with an aging population, we must look for new ways to ensure that older adults can contribute to and be cared for by their communities. The purpose of this paper is to provide an overview of research on planning and creating elder-friendly communities. First, we discuss the importance of the community environment to older persons and summarize research on older adults' definitions of community elder-friendliness. Next, we present a brief report of our own research on practitioners' definitions of elder-friendly community characteristics. Taken together, these definitions provide a platform for community efforts; however, because more specific guidelines are needed, we review tools to aid localities in becoming "age-prepared" by assessing their elder-friendliness and planning for future community needs. Finally we highlight strategies for developing elder-friendly communities using examples of local initiatives and review the implications for social workers.

THE COMMUNITY ENVIRONMENT AND OLDER PERSONS

Communities can support aging in place, but they may also contain barriers that make community living more difficult for older residents. Many homes and neighborhoods in which older people live were not designed for their changing needs and may present impediments to their well-being. Unless communities address issues of elder-friendliness, they may have to confront more aging-related problems in the future, such as a loss of older volunteers in community organizations, higher stress levels for family caregivers, and higher levels and costs of institutionalization. In order to remain active community participants, older adults may want accessible opportunities for involvement in community life and housing linked with or located near social activities and services. Additionally, as older persons aging in place experience declining capacity, they may need special transportation options, home modifications, in-home help, and other community-based services.

The future growth of the older population will necessitate a more integrated aging infrastructure, with increased housing, transportation, social service, and health care options that meet the needs of both active and frail older adults. Thus, developing elder-friendly communities to meet the needs of today's older adults and prepare for elders tomorrow is an issue of growing importance. Unfortunately, only a limited body of research exists to assist policymakers and practitioners in creating elder-friendly communities. Although there is a burgeoning planning literature (Norris, 2001) on the intersection between community design and quality of life (e.g., new urbanism, healthy communities, livable/walkable communities, smart growth), none of these community standards specifically addresses the needs of the nation's growing older population. For instance, although new urbanism addresses issues including housing density, mixed-use zoning, and walkability, it lacks emphasis on characteristics that may be more important to older persons, such as accessibility to community amenities, facilities, and services.

What Is an Elder-Friendly Community?

Currently, no uniform definition exists for the term "elder-friendly community." However, it generally refers to a place where older people are actively involved, valued, and supported with infrastructure and services that effectively accommodate their needs. This definition of elder-friendliness draws from the "person-environment fit" perspective (Lawton & Nahemow, 1973), which suggests that older adults must augment their capabilities when their individual levels of competence are challenged by the environment. This environment, which can be social, psychological, and/or physical, can either support or inhibit the capabilities and functioning of older persons. An elder-friendly community can moderate the demands of the environment and bring them in line with older individuals' strengths and deficits.

Because this conceptualization addresses the needs and competencies of older adults in a given area, elder-friendly communities vary in terms of emphasis. For instance, a rural community may require better transportation for service access, while an urban community may focus on walkability. An elder-friendly community, however, is not only for the retired or the frail; it provides a continuum of support for residents of all ages and all levels of ability. In essence, an elderly-friendly community makes local resources more "user-friendly" to older adults, so that services, programs, policies, and facilities maximize benefits to older adults and their families through convenience and support (Beier, 1997).

Older Adults' Definitions of Elder-Friendliness

Several studies have attempted to document the community characteristics that older adults identify as most important (Table 1). The largest investigation of older adults' opinions about their communities has been AARP's nationwide study of Americans over 45 (AARP, 2003). Participants were asked about both community characteristics and about those services most important to them in old age. At the local level, the City of Calgary (2001) and the Northwestern Illinois Area Agency on Aging (2002) conducted extensive focus groups of older adults and service providers in their respective catchment areas. In related research, 14 focus groups of older adults from around the country were assembled by the Center for Home Care Policy and Research to identify characteristics for aging in place (Feldman & Oberlink, 2003).

TABLE 1. Select Characteristics of Elder-Friendly Communities Identified by Older Persons

Study	AARP (2003)		City of Calgary (2001)	Northwestern Illinois (2000)	Feldman & Oberlink (2003)
Outcome	Characteristics of elder-friendliness	Services in elder-friendliness	Characteristics of elder-friendliness	Characteristics of elder-friendliness	Characteristics for aging in place
Characteristics of an elder-friendly community in order of importance	Safe neighborhoods	Door-to-door transportation	Seniors valued & respected	Transportation for seniors unable to drive	Financial security
	Hospital	Outdoor maintenance service	Opportunities to stay active	Affordable housing & housing alternatives	Health and health care
	Doctors' offices	Health monitoring service	Programs that build community & provide volunteer opportunities	Churches with an active social ministry outreach	Social connections
	Place to worship	Accessible public transportation	Services to help "make ends meet," (e.g., home repair services & affordable health care)	Senior organizations that provide both services and recreational programs	Housing and supportive services
	Shopping center	Home delivered meals	Safety, including home & community environment	A safe and caring community	Transportation and safety

The five most important factors identified by each study are reported in Table 1. Common elements across studies include transportation, housing, health care, safety, and respect for older community members; however, the relative importance of these items varies. Other critical aspects of the community environment included financial security and services to help "make ends meet," as well as an active social environment characterized by opportunities to stay active through both informal social networks and formal organizations.

Some of the variation across the studies may be the result of research focused on slightly different outcomes in different populations. Questions referring to elder-friendly services and characteristics necessary for aging in place produced responses more specifically relevant to frail older persons, such as the need for a health monitoring service or for housing with supportive services. In contrast, questions that more generally addressed elder-friendly neighborhoods highlighted the importance of social characteristics, such as active places of worship, recreational programs, and volunteer opportunities.

Practitioners' Perceptions of Elder-Friendliness

Clearly, older adults have a set of generally shared concerns and priorities regarding their communities, but little research has addressed whether practitioners understand and share these concerns. To address this issue, our research team conducted a study of fifteen national leaders in the fields of gerontology, urban planning, and community development, using the Delphi technique to develop a definition of elder-friendliness. The Delphi technique (Dalkey, 1969) is a method of generating ideas and facilitating consensus from the collective expertise of participants who are not necessarily in contact with each other. In a series of mail survey waves, participants first answer open-ended questions and then rate and reflect on responses, eventually producing a set of priorities based on numerical consensus.

Potential participants, including both researchers and practitioners, were identified based on an extensive literature review. Participants were first asked to respond to three open-ended questions, including: how to define an elder-friendly community; which are the most important characteristics in a community that would be considered elder-friendly; and what are potential examples of elder-friendly communities. From these open-ended questions, we assembled 39 community characteristics in five areas: service-oriented characteristics, such as meal sites and employment opportunities; physical community characteristics, such as accessible public buildings and streets designed for senior walking and driving; age-based services, such as senior centers and door-to-door transportation; community inclusiveness, such as opportunities for social integration and consideration of elders as vital citizens; and age-related infrastructure, such as elder-relevant issues present on the local agenda.

In the second and third waves of the study, participants were asked to rate and rank these characteristics in an effort to develop a concise set of community priorities. In this way, we were able to develop consensus among participants from different fields about the most important characteristics of an elder-friendly community. Table 2 shows the final results from the third wave.

Interestingly, many of these important community characteristics were the same as those identified by older adults. Community characteristics such as safety, a recognition of elders as an important part of the community, and accessible services were characterized as important by both practitioners and older adults. However, the researchers and practitioners who participated in the Delphi study also identified several more specific programs and environmental issues not identified by older persons as components of an elder-friendly community. For instance, Delphi study results highlight the need for caregiver support services and age-appropriate exercise facilities, perhaps reflecting the importance recent research and practice have placed on mental and physical health. Additionally, these results draw attention to the importance of the neighborhood physical environment, including characteristics such as supportive zoning for senior housing and adequate pedestrian and traffic controls.

ASSESSING ELDER-FRIENDLINESS
AND BECOMING AGE-PREPARED

Elder-friendly community definitions from both older adults and practitioners provide a platform for community efforts to serve the needs of older

TABLE 2. Elder-Friendly Community Characteristics: Delphi Study, 2002

Accessible and affordable transportation
Available in-home or long-term care services
A wide variety of appropriate housing options
Responsive health and long-term care
Ability to obtain services with reasonable travel
Personal safety and low crime rates
Elders considered vital part of community
Caregiver support services
Accessible public and service buildings
Elder-relevant issues present in local agenda
Recognition of and response to unique needs of seniors
A wide selection of services
Adequate pedestrian and traffic controls
Supportive zoning for senior housing
Age-appropriate exercise facilities

residents. However, communities may need more specific tools to assess their current neighborhood environments and to plan for the needs of future older persons. Becoming elder-friendly often requires not only addressing the needs of the current older population, but also planning for the needs of future older residents. An "age-prepared" community is one that has assessed its current services for older people and has planned for the needs of its future older population. Communities can and do work toward elder-friendliness by becoming age-prepared, assessing current resources and projecting future needs, then responding to these needs through planning. Because the needs and resources of older adults vary by community, this process will also vary. Thus, community assessments represent an important starting place in becoming age-prepared.

Needs Assessments

The term "needs assessment" refers to a broad array of activities designed to determine the discrepancy between what is available and what should be (Posavac & Carey, 1997). Appropriate assessment is a key element of social work, case management, and community practice. Community organizations and planning departments often conduct a needs assessment to develop new programs or to expand, refine, or improve existing programs.

Both qualitative approaches, such as focus groups or in-depth client interviews, and quantitative approaches, such as surveys of target groups, can be useful. However, these two methods require different levels of investment and provide different types of information (Kunkel, 2003). Qualitative approaches yield rich insights about needs and services that may be useful in designing interventions. They can yield detailed information about targeted groups, such as older persons with disabilities, senior center users, or residents of a particular neighborhood. In general, they tend to require a smaller investment in research, because they typically utilize fewer participants.

In contrast, quantitative approaches may be most useful when some information is already available in the process of planning future programs or expanding services. They can help address questions related to program planning, such as "how many people think this is a problem?" or "where do most community residents who need services live?" Quantitative approaches often require a substantial investment of time and funds because of the requirements of survey design and data collection for a representative survey, whether data collection occurs through mail surveys, phone surveys, or face-to-face interviews. One strategy for accomplishing this type of assessment is to form a coalition of interested parties, such as the local planning department, Area Agency on Aging, Public Housing Authority, and municipal or regional transit agency, as well as agencies that serve seniors. All these groups are likely to have some interest in a community survey for their own specific purposes, and they may be able to contribute to its development and implementation.

Elder-Friendly Community Assessments

As older adults, researchers, and practitioners have recognized the importance of creating elder-friendly communities, they have also realized the need for more specific indicators of elder-friendliness for use in needs assessments. In response to this need, several assessments have been created that address a wide variety of community characteristics. They include the AARP Livable Communities Guide (Pollak, 1999), the AdvantAge Initiative (Feldman & Oberlink, 2003), and the Elder Ready Community Report Cards (Hernandez, 2001a, 2001b) used in Florida. Each emphasizes the importance of community involvement in conducting the assessment and includes indicators relevant to community services, the private sector, and the built environment.

The AARP Livable Communities Guide (Pollak, 1999) is perhaps the most extensive, with 100 specific questions on topics ranging from affordable housing to community recreation centers. Although designed to address the needs of older adults, this guide pertains to age-related issues that affect all community residents. However, because it relies exclusively on presence or absence measures, it has a limited ability to address issues such as affordability and accessibility of available services.

In Florida, Hernandez (2001a, 2001b) has developed a system of report cards, including the *Access Ready Report Card for Well Elders* and the *Elder Ready Community Report Card for Frail Elders*. These assessments independently address needs applicable to independent older persons (e.g., driving, accessible shopping) and those relevant to frail older persons (e.g., home care, assisted living). Compared to other assessments, these report cards place greater emphasis on non-governmental organizations, including businesses and places of worship. However, like the AARP assessment, they are made up almost exclusively of presence or absence measures, with little emphasis on affordability and accessibility.

The AdvantAge Initiative (Feldman & Oberlink, 2003, p. 273) presents a concise list of 33 essential elements of an elder-friendly community, including items such as "percentage of people age 65 + who want to remain in their current residence and are confident they will be able to afford to do so" and "percentage of people age 65 + who participate in volunteer work." This assessment is specific to older adults, and is unique in that it focuses on both basic needs (e.g., housing, meals, personal care) and on maximizing independence and community involvement. Furthermore, in contrast to the AARP assessment, the AdvantAge tool incorporates need as well as availability of services.

Both the AARP and Florida assessments consist of flexible questions that could be used in qualitative focus groups or a quantitative survey method. However, as noted above, they are limited in their ability to identify specific needs. In contrast, the AdvantAge Initiative focuses extensively on identifying unmet needs relative to current resources. Because this assessment emphasizes the prevalence of problems among older adults in the community, it necessitates a more quantitative approach with a random sampling of community members; this approach is likely to yield data useful for planning and implementing a variety of community programs.

DEVELOPING ELDER-FRIENDLY COMMUNITIES: LOCAL INITIATIVES

In the past, policy initiatives have emphasized specific institutions and services such as health care and, to a lesser extent, housing. However, several forces are driving communities to engage in new initiatives that utilize assessments like those above and span different policy domains to support life in the community. These forces include population aging, a renewed focus on self-determination and individual responsibility, and the implementation of the Olmstead decision, which requires states to plan for less restrictive options for persons with disabilities (O'Hara & Day, 2001). Building elder-friendly communities requires a more integrated perspective that coordinates health, housing, and transportation services and bridges the gap between social services and the built environments. Creating policies that encourage elder-friendly community planning and development requires a paradigm shift, integrating the aging network with the disability network, bringing planners and service providers together, and opening and sustaining dialogues between public agencies and private businesses.

Community Examples

Available examples from local initiatives demonstrate the importance of having a lead organization to convene stakeholders, conduct assessments, and provide continuity throughout the process of implementing initiatives. For instance, the "Coming of Age in Rural Illinois" project was sponsored by Illinois State University. Researchers were able to use existing data from the Illinois Rural Life Panel Survey to inform their understanding of community needs and to build on this survey using new data from key informants in local government, law enforcement, health care, and senior services (Beier, 1997). The "A Place to Call Home" project in Calgary was a partnership between the City of Calgary, the Calgary Regional Health Authority, and the faculty of Social Work at the University of Calgary (City of Calgary, 2001).

Such research-practitioner partnerships match university research skills in needs assessment with community practitioners' and stakeholders' abilities to turn results into programs and services. Smaller efforts have also benefited from such partnerships. For instance, at a NORC (naturally occurring retirement community) site in Los Angeles, the Jewish Family Services, a local service provider, is working with aging researchers and a wide range of community groups to create an environment more friendly to area resident needs. In a related community effort, researchers conducted a study of a busy neighborhood intersection and found that older pedestrians had difficulty crossing (Hoxie & Rubinstein, 1994). Based on these findings, service providers successfully lobbied the city transportation department for increased crossing time, thereby improving intersection safety.

Leadership and continuity can also come from a variety of community non-profit or religious organizations. For instance, the Evergreen Institute in Bloomington, Indiana is a community non-profit organization dedicated to promoting a healthy urban environment for older adults by creating neighborliness, diverse housing options, and intergenerational programs. The Institute's programs were guided by an initial telephone survey of older residents that addressed neighborhood issues including housing, health care needs, retail and social services, and safety issues. Such surveys can form the basis of an integrated approach that addresses comprehensive community change.

Finally, in an example that suggests the power of long-term planning, the City of Pasadena has succeeded, by many of the indicators mentioned previously, in creating an elder-friendly community for its more than 15,000 older residents. This development occurred through conscientious planning that addressed both age-based and age-related issues in a variety of city agencies and community organizations. In 1995, the city created a Master Plan for Seniors that provides information on senior needs, services, and policy recommendations through the Year 2005. The purpose of the plan was to "analyze local demographics, assess the needs in the community, and to identify resources, duplications and gaps in services" (City of Pasadena, 1995, p. 9).

The City Human Services and Neighborhoods Department began the planning process by creating a Senior Master Plan Committee that was designed to be as inclusive and open as possible. The committee was composed of individuals, local community leaders, agency representatives, and city employees from several departments. It gathered demographic data from the 1990 census and compiled information from previous assessments, including general community assessments (e.g., the 1995 Pasadena Citizens Survey, surveys by the Community Health Alliance of Pasadena), as well as assessments specific to older persons (e.g., a recent assessment of Latino elderly). The committee received input from every agency in the city and hosted several public forums in different parts of the city to receive input on issues related to seniors.

In its final form, the master plan outlined unmet needs and available ser-·vices in areas including case management, employment, grandparenting, health care, housing, legal assistance, mental health, in-home services, transportation, and volunteer opportunities. Recommendations based on these findings were organized by one-year, five-year, and ten-year goals. Outcomes of the plan include a directory of senior programs and services and creation of a Senior Advocacy Council. Additionally, the plan has helped the Pasadena Senior Center expand service offerings and establish satellite programs in community centers around Pasadena, serving more residents near their homes. This example illustrates how a network of interested agencies and organizations can build upon existing assessments with qualitative research to create a long-range impact on the community.

Implications for Social Work

A focus on elder-friendly communities can be seen as the natural outgrowth of an increase in the older population and the on-going shift toward a community orientation in gerontological social work. In the last decade, the field of social work has witnessed an enormous growth in the emphasis on community, with the expansion of case management and community practice. Case management entails "a procedure to plan, seek, and monitor services from different social agencies and staff on behalf of a client" (Barker, 2003, p. 58). Consequently, case managers require a thorough knowledge of community resources that allow older clients to remain in the least restrictive environment possible. At the same time, community practice requires "the application of practice skills to alter the behavioral patterns of community groups, organizations, and institutions or people's relationships and interactions with these entities" (Hardcastle, Wenocur, & Powers, 1997, p. 399). From the community practice perspective, communities act as systems composed of subsystems such as mental health and social services. Social workers involved in community practice help to ensure that these systems are functional for clients (Hardcastle, Wenocur, & Powers, 1997). A community focus may require social workers to create new partnerships with planners and policymakers to pursue broader community goals for the support of older persons. Communities can and must develop cohesive local strategies to address the issues of an aging population, in which localities and community organizations respond to resident needs, advocate for appropriate service provision, and plan for supportive environments for their future elders.

Implications for Practice

Across all the studies and initiatives described above, two general themes emerge. First, results indicate the importance of *age-based* community issues, or those programs and services specifically intended to address the needs of older persons, as well as *age-related* community issues, or those programs and services from which older persons may benefit, but that address issues relevant to the broader community or to specific subgroups, such as disabled or dependent residents (e.g., children) or minority groups. (For a discussion of these differences, see Hudson, 1995.) For instance, age-based community services include senior programs, such as exercise or volunteering designed exclusively for older adults, as well as programs designed to meet the needs of special groups, including disabled older persons and their caregivers. In contrast, age-related community issues include the need for accessible public transportation, nearby doctors and shopping centers, and safe neighborhoods. While these community features may be particularly crucial for improving older persons' quality of life, they are likely to be important to all community residents, regardless of age.

Recognizing this distinction is important, because it can help social workers in community practice identify key stakeholders when advocating for elder-friendly programs and services. For instance, expanding the availability of caregiver support services, a predominantly age-based service, will probably mean working with local senior centers, home care agencies, and age-based consumer groups. In contrast, addressing an age-related community characteristic, such as the creation of safer pedestrian and traffic controls, may mean working with transportation planners, citizen organizations, and neighborhood block groups.

A second theme evident from existing research on elder-friendly communities is the importance of both the *social* environment and the *built* environment, as well as the relationship between them, reflecting environmental press. For instance, safety and other social factors, such as a community's respect for older adults and available opportunities to stay active, contribute significantly to older adults' quality of life. At the same time, the importance of the neighborhood built environment is evident in the need for accessible public and service buildings, services available within reasonable travel time, availability of sidewalks or other pedestrian safety measures, and affordable housing and zoning supportive of senior housing.

The social and built environments represent important areas for community-practice advocacy and interventions. Because changes in the built environment can require years to enact, planning is an essential part of creating change in community environments. Planning makes a difference in how services are delivered and how clients access them. For instance, if a senior center is located near residents' homes or public transit routes, older persons will have better access to services. In contrast, a lack of planning that integrates the physical and social environments can make service delivery more difficult. This problem exists in many Section 202 buildings, a type of affordable housing for the elderly, which have been built without public space; these buildings now require extensive retrofitting to provide aging residents with needed meal programs and services (Heumann, Winter-Nelson, & Anderson, 2001). These examples illustrate the interplay between the social and built environments.

Unfortunately, older citizens are often left out of the plan-making process, and community plans may not adequately consider the needs of older residents (Boswell, 2000). Social workers can address the built environment by helping older people identify their concerns about housing, transportation, and zoning issues and empowering them to present their views in appropriate forums, such as planning meetings and zoning hearings. Additionally, social workers can work more directly with planners to represent their clients' concerns. In this way, they can help reduce fragmentation and create environments that better serve older adults. Figure 1 displays some key terms and resources from urban planning that may be useful for social workers and community practitioners in developing elder-friendly communities and working with planners.

CONCLUSION

Increasingly, a variety of stakeholders recognize the importance of creating elder-friendly communities, including older consumers, community planners, and aging service providers. Social workers are in a unique position to contribute to such community efforts, because they are likely to be familiar with community needs and resources and have established contacts with a variety of organizations. Furthermore, social workers stand to benefit from the development of elder-friendly communities, because they will be better able to help older clients in a more supportive community. Social workers and other service providers can reap professional rewards from creating new relationships with planners and policymakers to prepare communities for the future and to develop elder-friendly communities.

Some community characteristics, such as accessible and affordable transportation, housing, and health care, as well as safety and opportunities for community involvement, have emerged from research as crucial to older adults' ability to age in the community. However, the specific nature and priority of these issues vary according to an individual community's current capacity and

FIGURE 1. Key Terms and Resources for Planning Elder-Friendly Communities

Accessibility: Consistent with the Americans with Disabilities Act (ADA), public entities including businesses and services must be designed in a way that permits their use by persons with disabilities
  Department of Justice ADA: www.ada.gov

Built environment: Those aspects of our environment that are human modified such as homes, schools, workplaces, parks, industrial areas, farms, roads and highways
  National Institute of Environmental Health Sciences: www.niehs.nih.gov

Healthy communities: Movement to create communities that promote and sustain health by creating a positive physical environment, a vital economy, and a supportive social climate
  International Healthy Cities Foundation: www.healthycities.org
  Healthy people 2010: www.healthypeople.gov

Livable communities: Movement to promote smart growth and new urbanism through creating mixed-use development in which people live, work, and play in clean, safe neighborhoods with a decreased reliance on automobile travel
  Local Government Commission Center for Livable Communities:
   www.lgc.org/center
  American Institute of Architects: www.aia.org/livable

New urbanism: Focus on urban planning that is pedestrian-focused, including new development, redevelopment, and in-fill development that aim to produce walkable neighborhoods that include a mix of housing and jobs
  Congress for New Urbanism: www.cnu.org

Smart growth: Smart growth involves investing time, attention, and resources in restoring community and promoting vitality in center cities and older suburbs. New smart growth is town-centered, transit and pedestrian oriented, and utilizes a greater mix of housing, commercial and retail uses
  Smart Growth Network: www.smartgrowth.org

Universal design: Universal design is the design of products and environments to be usable by all people, to the greatest extent possible, without the need for adaptation or specialized design
  Center for Universal Design: www.design.ncsu.edu/cud

Visitability: Movement to create single family homes that are "visitable" by persons with disabilities, including a minimum of a zero-step entrance, 32-inch doors, and a bathroom on the main floor
  Concrete Change: www.concretechange.org

Walkable communities: Movement to help communities become more walkable and pedestrian friendly, with the premise that walkable communities put urban environments back on a scale for sustainability of resources (both natural and economic) and lead to more social interaction, physical fitness and diminished crime and other social problems
  Walkable Communities, Inc: www.walkable.org

its older population's needs. Thus, a community needs assessment is an important beginning to becoming age-prepared, and social workers can be instrumental in contributing to this process. Given limited resources, they can also use the results to determine which community needs are most urgent and which characteristics are most amenable to social work intervention.

Even in communities where a needs assessment is not available or not feasible, social workers can be involved in making a community more elder-friendly. Social workers can and should be involved in the implementation of new programs and community initiatives to advocate for their clients. For instance, community practitioners can participate in the creation of a local Consolidated Plan, advocating for more affordable senior housing or for more services in existing housing. They can act as community change agents, encouraging city agencies to conduct hearings in areas that are accessible to older adults, or appearing themselves at public meetings, including city council and zoning meetings, to represent the concerns of older community members. Even more important, they can encourage and empower their clients to advocate for their own needs and provide direct input into community assessment and planning processes.

The Future

In the future, more research on older adults in the community should address the process of becoming elder-friendly, with a focus on identifying the most effective strategies for use by social workers and other practitioners. Research should address ways of incorporating the goals of elder-friendly communities into policy measures, such as the community General Plan. Furthermore, outcomes-related research is needed at the individual level to assess the importance of elder-friendly communities. For instance, we must ask how community interventions affect the quality of life of older persons. Which interventions are most important to support aging in place? How can we best meet the needs of the diverse elderly of the future, including both the well and frail elderly? How can community-level interventions impact the quality of life of vulnerable populations, including low-income, rural, and minority older persons? These questions will be even more important in the future, necessitating a response from both research and practice today.

REFERENCES

AARP. (2000). *Fixing to stay: A national survey on housing and home modification issues.* Washington DC: Author.

AARP. (2003). *These four walls: Americans 45 + talk about home and community.* Washington, DC: Author.

Barker, R. L. (2003). *The social work dictionary.* 5th ed. Washington, DC: NASW Press.

Beier, L. M. (1997). *Coming of age in rural Illinois: Developing elder-friendly communities.* Normal, IL: Illinois State University. Retrieved December 12, 2003, from http://www.asru.ilstu.edu/reports/RRFfinrpt.PDF.

Boswell, D. (2000). *Older citizens and the plan-making process: Are planners being neglectful?* (Working Paper No. 69). University of New Orleans, Division of Urban Research and Policy Studies.

City of Calgary. (2001). *A place to call home: Final report of the elder-friendly communities project.* Calgary, Alberta: University of Calgary. Retrieved September 15, 2003 from http://www.calgary.ca/docgallery/BU/community/elder_friendly_com munities.pdf.

City of Pasadena. (1995). *Master plan for seniors: Needs, services, and policy recommendations through the Year 2005.* Pasadena, CA: Author.

Dalkey, N. (1969). *The Delphi method: An experimental study of group opinion.* Santa Monica, CA: RAND Corporation.

Feldman, P. H., & Oberlink, M. R. (2003). The AdvantAge Initiative: Developing community indicators to promote the health and well-being of older people. *Family and Community Health, 26*, 268-274.

Feldman, P. H., Oberlink, M. R., Simantov, E., & Gursen, M. D. (2004). *A tale of two older Americas: Community opportunities and challenges.* New York: Center for Home Care Policy and Research. Retrieved May 18, 2004 from http://www.vnsny.org/advantage/AI_NationalSurveyReport.pdf.

Hardcastle, D., Wenocur, S., & Powers, P. (1997). *Community practice: Theories and skills for social workers.* Pacific Grove, CA: Brooks/Cole.

Hernandez, G. (2001a). *Elder ready community report card for frail elders.* Tallahassee, FL: Florida Department of Elder Affairs.

Hernandez, G. (2001b). *Report card for well elders.* Tallahassee, FL: Communities for Life.

Heumann, L., Winter-Nelson, K., & Anderson, J. (2001). *The 1999 National Housing Survey of Section 202 Elderly Housing* (#2001-02). Washington, DC: AARP.

Hoxie, R. E., & Rubinstein, L. Z. (1994). Are older pedestrians allowed enough time to cross intersections safely? *Journal of the American Geriatrics Society, 42, 1219-1220.*

Hudson, R. B. (1995). The history and place of age-based public policy. *Generations, 14*(3), 5-10.

Kinsella, K., & Velkoff, V. A. (2001). *An aging world: 2001* (U.S. Census Bureau, Series P95/01-1). Washington, DC: U.S. Government Printing Office.

Kunkel, S. (2003). Assessing community needs. *Center for Medicare Education Issue Brief, 4,* 1-6.

Lawton, M. P., & Nahemow, L. (1973). Ecology and the aging process. In C. Eisdorfer & M. P. Lawton (Eds.) *Psychology of adult development.* Washington, DC: American Psychological Association.

Norris, T. (2001). America's communities movement: Investing in the civic landscape. *American Journal of Community Psychology, 29,* 301-308.

Northwestern Illinois Area Agency on Aging. (2000). *Creating elder-friendly communities.* Rockford, IL: Author.

O'Hara, A., & Day, S. (2001). *Olmstead and supportive housing: A vision for the future.* Princeton, NJ: Center for Health Care Strategies.

Pollak, P. B. (1999). *Liveable communities: An evaluation guide.* Washington, DC: AARP.

Posavac, E. J., & Carey, R. G. (1997). *Program evaluation: Methods and case studies.* 5th ed. Englewood Cliffs, NJ: Prentice Hall.

Pynoos, J. (1993). Strategies for home modification and repair. In J. Callahan (Ed.), *Aging in place* (pp. 29-38). Amityville, NY: Baywood.

U.S. Administration on Aging (2003). *A profile of older Americans: 2003.* Washington, DC: Administration on Aging. Retrieved February 21, 2004 from http://www.aoa.gov/prof/Statistics/profile/2003/profiles2003.asp.

doi:10.1300/J083v49n01_01

Living on the Margins:
Older Homeless Adults in Toronto

Lynn McDonald, PhD
Julie Dergal, MSc
Laura Cleghorn, MA

SUMMARY. A handful of scholars have acknowledged that, along side the traditional homeless, there are now older people who become homeless for the first time in old age. Few researchers, however, have systematically compared the recent older homeless with the chronic or traditional homeless. In the research presented here, we compare recent older homeless with long-term older homeless adults in Toronto according to their health and wealth, their housing history, and their use of health and social services. Findings indicate that people who become homeless for the first time at older ages have needs that are different from the lifetime elderly homeless and require different approaches to intervention. doi:10.1300/ J083v49n01_02 *[Article copies available for a fee from The Haworth Document Delivery Service: 1-800-HAWORTH. E-mail address: <docdelivery@haworth press.com> Website: <http://www.HaworthPress.com> © 2007 by The Haworth Press, Inc. All rights reserved.]*

KEYWORDS. Older homeless, chronic homeless, long-term homeless, new homeless

---

[Haworth co-indexing entry note]: "Living on the Margins: Older Homeless Adults in Toronto." McDonald, Lynn, Julie Dergal, and Laura Cleghorn. Co-published simultaneously in *Journal of Gerontological Social Work* (The Haworth Press, Inc.) Vol. 49, No. 1/2, 2007, pp. 19-46; and: *Housing for the Elderly: Policy and Practice Issues* (ed: Philip McCallion) The Haworth Press, Inc., 2007, pp. 19-46. Single or multiple copies of this article are available for a fee from The Haworth Document Delivery Service [1-800-HAWORTH, 9:00 a.m. - 5:00 p.m. (EST). E-mail address: docdelivery@haworthpress.com].

INTRODUCTION

Gerontological social workers have long been committed to maximizing housing options for older adults, even in the face of dwindling low-cost housing (Burnette, Morrow-Howell, & Chen, 2003; Council of Social Work Education, 2001). It is therefore ironic that just as social workers become accustomed to helping older clients "age-in-place" they are confronted with a growing sub-population of older adults who literally do not have a place. While there is a small but growing body of research on older homeless adults that began in the mid 1980s, the available evidence about their problems and needs and the services to meet these needs is slim and sometimes contradictory. In particular, the literature pays little attention to the heterogeneity of the older homeless population although there have been some attempts to distinguish the young from the older homeless (Gelberg, Linn, & Meyer-Oakes, 1990; Hallebone, 1997; Hecht & Coyle, 2001) and older homeless women from older homeless men (Cohen, Ramirez, Teresi, Gallagher & Sokolovsky, 1997; Kutza & Keigher, 1991; Stergiopoulos & Herrmann, 2003). There also have been attempts to study a narrow range of characteristics of older homeless adults such as whether they are veterans (Applewhite, 1997; Bruckner, 2001), American Indians (Kramer & Barker, 1996); African Americans (Killion, 2000), or suffer from mental illness (Auslander & Jeste, 2002; Cohen, Onserud & Monaco, 1992; DeMallie, North & Smith, 1997; Fisher, Turner, Pugh & Taylor, 1994).

A handful of scholars have acknowledged that, along side the traditional older homeless–the stereotypical tramp-like figures who choose to be homeless–there are now older people who become homeless for the first time in old age (Cohen & Sokolovsky, 1989; Crane, 1994; O'Connell, Summerfield, Kellogg, 1990; O'Reilly-Flemming, 1993). Few researchers, however, have systematically compared the new older homeless with the chronic or traditional homeless other than to note their presence in passing (Crane & Warnes, 2001; Doolin, 1986; Morbey, Pannell & Means, 2003; Rosenheck & Seibyl, 1998). In the research presented here, we compare the new older homeless with long-term older homeless adults according to their health and wealth, their housing history, and their use of health and social services. The comparison is made because it is hypothesized that people who become homeless for the first time at older ages may have needs that are different from the lifetime elderly homeless.

THE EXTENT OF HOMELESSNESS AMONG OLDER ADULTS

The exact number of older homeless adults and their share of the homeless population are not easily verified for a host of complex reasons. Because homelessness tends to be episodic with a constant flow of people between housed and homeless states, it has been difficult to obtain accurate prevalence and incidence data (Piliavin, Wright, Mare & Westerfelt, 1996; Wong, Culhane & Kuhn, 1997). As a result, the number of people who are homeless at a particular time is only a fraction of those who are ever homeless (Crane, 1996). To complicate matters further, investigations of the homeless use a wide variety of definitions of homelessness (Cohen, 1999); the age at which someone is labeled old varies anywhere from age 40 to 65 (Cohen, 1999; Crane & Warnes, 2001; Stergiopoulos & Herrmann, 2003), and older homeless people are very difficult to identify and therefore hard to find (Crane, 1996; Rossi, 1989; Vance, 1994). Possibly because of the relative neglect of older homeless adults by researchers, not all data on homelessness include statistics on the proportion of older adults in their sample (DeMallie et al., 1997; Gibeau, 2001).

Overall, most homeless estimates are highly variable and are reported to span anywhere from 2 to 27% of the homeless population for those over 50 years of age (Burt, 1992; Cohen, 1999; Crane & Warnes, 2000; Crane & Warnes, 2001; Rosenheck, Bassuk & Salomon, 1999). It has been estimated that between 60,000 and 400,000 older people are currently homeless in the United States and these numbers are increasing in absolute terms due to the aging of the baby boom population.[1] A recent report by the Canadian Mortgage and Housing Corporation summarizes existing data from major cities and found that from 5 to 9% of shelter users were 55 years of age and over (Serge & Gnaedinger, 2003). In a Toronto study, 10% of shelter users were over age 50 (Springer, Mars, & Dennison, 1998) while the Canadian Census data indicated that 10% of shelter users for all of Canada were 65 years of age and over (Statistics Canada, 2002).

Despite the uncertainty about the numbers of older homeless adults, there is little doubt that the population will increase as the baby boom generation ages, particularly if affordable housing continues to remain in short supply (British Columbia Ministry of Social Development and Economic Security, 2001; Crane & Warnes, 2001; Doolin, 1986; Hecht & Coyle, 2001; Keigher & Greenblatt, 1992; Rosenheck et al., 1999; Tully & Jacobson, 1994). In the United States, for example, Cohen (1999) predicts, that with the aging of the baby boomers, the older homeless population will grow to between 120,000 to 800,000 over the next three decades. Once older people become homeless, they have a more difficult time improving their circumstances. Research suggests that the average length of homelessness is higher among older homeless people, and higher among men than women (Hecht & Coyle, 2001; North & Smith, 1993; Roth, Tomey, & First, 1992).

These demographic shifts portend a greater need for social workers to support the older homeless and to help them navigate increasingly complex health and social services programs. As the *Blueprint* by the Council on Social Work

Education notes, "The rapid increase in older adults ... suggests that ALL social workers should have basic competence in aging" (Council of Social Work Education, 2001, p. v). From our perspective, the *Blueprint* would include those working with elderly homeless persons. As one older recently homeless woman in our study noted, "I find there is nothing really for our age . . . we're . . . baby boomers, the forgotten baby boomers."

THE CAUSES OF THE HOMELESSNESS OF OLDER ADULTS

The discourse about the root causes of homelessness of older persons is long on conjecture and short on evidence. The proposed causes do not appear to be much different than what is offered in the broader homeless literature. Briefly, explanations focus on structural issues that are often beyond the control of the individual (Avramov, 1995; Greve, 1991; Wolch, Dear, & Akita, 1988), and personal vulnerabilities that jeopardize an individual's capacity to maintain stable housing (Hecht & Coyle, 2001). Usually both sets of causes are seen to interact pushing a person into homelessness, sometimes with a specific event acting as a trigger (Cohen, 1999; Crane & Warnes, 2001). For example, Hallebone (1997) in Australia relies more on the structural factors when she cites the retrenchment of the welfare state, the shortage of government-subsidized rental housing, and the decline in affordable housing as the main causes of homelessness amongst the young and the old. These views are echoed by Bottomley, Bissonette, and Snekvik (2001) and Rosenheck et al. (1999) in the United States, while Hecht and Coyle (2001) argue that access to affordable housing is the root cause of homelessness, especially for minorities. Deinstitutionalization of mental health patients and poverty are also seen to be major structural causative factors (Rosenheck et al., 1999; Tully & Jacobson, 1994). Alcohol and substance abuse problems, family breakdown, and health problems would be examples of individual factors (Wright, Rubin, & Devine, 1998).

Although studies have failed to examine the differences between homelessness for people who have been homeless for many years, and those who have become homeless in later life (Crane, 1996) factors such as eviction, marital breakdown (loss of a spouse), retirement and loss of income, and widowhood have been commonly cited as reasons for homelessness at older ages (Crane, 1996; Crane & Warnes, 2001). A model for homelessness and aging that combines structural and individual factors has been recently proposed (Cohen, 1999) and suggests that risk factors for being homeless accumulate over a lifetime, and that homelessness is not likely to occur unless several factors co-exist. It has been suggested that homelessness among women is more likely to stem from family crises (e.g., marital breakdown, widowhood), while for men, it is often work-related challenges (e.g., loss of employment) (Cohen, 1999).

In terms of our interest in the differences between long-term and recent homelessness at older ages, both Crane and Warnes (2000) and Rosenheck et al. (1999) have made some preliminary observations. In a study of 267 older homeless adults in the United Kingdom, Crane and Warnes (2000) found three pathways into homelessness: people who were homeless since adolescence because of broken homes, army discharge, or marital breakdown; middle-aged adults who had lived with parents who died and who could not cope on their own after their death; people who became homeless in old age because of widowhood, marital breakdown, or mental illness (Crane & Warnes, 2000). Rosenheck et al. (1999), in a review of the research in the U.S., found that older persons became homeless because of the death of a spouse or caretaker.

THE UNIQUE CHARACTERISTICS OF OLDER HOMELESS ADULTS

Older persons without a home are of special concern because of their vulnerability to victimization, their frailty due to poor mental and physical health, and the reluctance of traditional aging services to incorporate them into programs (Bottomly et al., 2001; Kutza & Keigher, 1991; Morbey et al., 2003; Roberstson & Greenblatt, 1992; Serge & Gnaedinger, 2003; Vermette, 1994). Harsh living conditions exacerbate their acute and chronic health problems so that older homeless people appear older than those of the same age living in stable housing. The following is an overview of what is more commonly known about older homeless adults at this time.

Age

A number of researchers have found evidence that there should be a lower age threshold for defining old because many homeless adults appear and behave 10 to 20 years older than the general population (Crane & Warnes, 2000; Cohen, 1999) and their life expectancy is lower (Crane & Warnes, 2001). The research indicates that mortality rates are higher for older homeless adults and they are more likely to die from preventable diseases and accidental/unintentional injury like freezing to death (Ashe, Brandon, Contogouris, & Swanson, 1996; Barrow, Herman, Cordova, & Struening, 1999; Hibbs, Benne, Klugman, Spencer, Macchia, & Mellinger et al., 1994; Hwang, Orav, O'Connell, Lebow, & Brennan, 1997; Hwang, 2000; Hwang, O'Connell, Lebow, Bierer, Orav, & Brennan, 2001). For example, in the United States, age-adjusted mortality rates among the homeless in a study in Philadelphia was 3.5 times that for

Philadelphia's general population (Hibbs et al., 1994) and in New York 4 times the rate of the general population (Barrow et al., 1999). In contrast, in Toronto, mortality rates for men aged 45 to 64 were twice that for men in the general population (Hwang et al., 2001), possibly because of a lower incidence of homicide in Canada. Whatever the figures, it has been stated that "one of the costs of being homeless in the America is losing about 20 years of life expectancy" (Wright, Rubin, & Devine, 1998, p. 167).

Gender

The gender division in the homeless population is different from the general population, where the numbers of women outnumber men (Cohen, 1999). Among the aging homeless population, however, the reverse is true. In addition, the patterns of homelessness are different for men and women. Studies from the United States and the United Kingdom have shown that men have been homeless about 50% longer than women (Crane & Warnes, 2000; Rossi, 1989), and that older women often become homeless for the first time in their mid-fifties (Cohen & Crane, 1996).

Social Support

The research suggests that older homeless people have social networks approximately three-fourths the size of the older general population. Research from the United States found that the networks of homeless people tend to include people from agencies and institutions, and to have fewer intimate ties (Cohen et al., 1997). U.S. studies of older homeless people found that less than 8% were currently married, less than 25% were widowed, between one-third and one-half were divorced or separated, and about one-fifth to one-third had never been married (Cohen & Crane, 1996; Gelberg et al., 1990; Roth et al., 1992). Compared to younger homeless people, older homeless people are isolated, they do not congregate on the streets with other homeless people, they appear more detached, and the majority have no or minimal contact with family members (Gelberg et al., 1990). Research has also shown that lack of perceived social support is a risk factor for homelessness (Cohen et al., 1997; Kisor & Kendal-Wilson, 2002).

Physical Health

In light of the higher mortality rates of older homeless adults, it comes as no surprise that their physical and mental health is poorer than the general older population. Homelessness increases a person's exposure to infectious and communicable diseases, the severe stress of the homeless experience can trigger genetic dispositions like hypertension, and long periods of malnutrition can cause some chronic conditions like anemia or degenerative bone disease. To make things worse, unacceptable living conditions also result in poor hygiene, inadequate diets, exposure to the elements, irregular sleep, and physical injuries (Eberle Planning and Research, 2002; Kushner, 1998).

A cohort study in Toronto of men, aged 45 to 64 using homeless shelters from 1995 to 1997, found that the main causes of death were: cancer, heart disease, cerebrovascular disease, and accidental deaths. With the exception of accidental deaths, these causes differed from younger age groups, where poisoning, suicide, and AIDS were the most common causes. Similar findings were reported in the United States. A cohort study of slightly more than 17,000 homeless adults seen by the Boston Health Care for the Homeless Program from 1988 to 1993 was conducted to obtain the causes of death among homeless people. Heart disease and cancer were the leading causes of death among those aged 45 to 64, which was different from younger groups (homicide, AIDS). For the entire cohort, the mean age of death was forty-seven. Death occurred most commonly in a hospital (54%), or in a residential setting (19%), while only 3% of the cohort died in a nursing home (Hwang et al., 1997).

Mental Health

There is a strong connection between homelessness and mental health and it is generally estimated that about one-third of homeless people suffer from mental illness. The rates of mental illness vary by subgroup and the older homeless are no exception. Although research is scant on older persons, a handful of studies indicate significant psychiatric morbidity in this population (Abdul-Hamid, 1997; Acorn, 1993; Cohen & Sokolovsky, 1989; Crane & Warnes, 2001; DeMallie et al., 1997; Gelberg et al., 1990; Ladner, 1992). For example, Cohen, Tresi, Holmes, and Roth (1988) in their study of older homeless men in New York, used non-diagnostic scales to discover that one-third of the men were clinically depressed and 23% were psychotic. In an overview of studies, Stergiopoulos and Hermann (2003) uncovered depression, psychosis, and cognitive impairment as the specific psychiatric disorders cited most frequently for older homeless people. In a recent study in Australia, the prevalence of cognitive impairment among men and women with an average age of 57 years was 10% as assessed by the Mini Mental State Examination (Buhrich, Hodder & Teeson, 2000). Compared with men, a greater proportion of older homeless women have poor mental health (Crane & Warnes, 2000; Eberle, 2000; Rosenheck et al., 1999). According to Crane and Warnes (2000), in London hostels mental illness rose with age and the biggest increase was for women, jumping from 5 to 10% of women under 20 years of age to 57% of those aged 50 to 59 and 76% of those aged 60 and over.

Substance Abuse

Added to these physical and mental health problems is the problem of alcohol abuse which is three or four times more prevalent among older homeless men than women (Fischer & Breakey, 1991); reportedly increases with age (Kershaw, Singleton, & Meltzer, 2000) and the rates for either gender are higher compared to the general older population (Ladner, 1992). The literature suggests both survivor and cohort effects. That is, as homeless people age, those with higher alcohol abuse levels tend to die or are unable to live in shelters or on the streets and may be placed in long-term care or congregate living arrangements. Higher rates of lifetime histories of alcohol abuse among those aged 50 and over have been found, while drug use is more common among the younger homeless. To date, illicit drug use tends not to be common among older homeless people, possibly because there may be a generation effect (Cohen, 1999). That is, the rates of use and/or abuse may be higher for those born between 1946 and 1964, or the generation that followed. Some research suggests that older homeless people may not have escaped the cocaine era (DeMallie et al., 1997).

Recent studies of alcohol and drug patterns among older homeless adults are limited (Boucher, 1995). A few studies report alcohol problems ranging from 30 to 37% among those aged 50 to 64, and from 1 to 18% among those aged 65 and over. Alcoholism is difficult to diagnose among older adults and may be easily overlooked or attributed to physiological changes of aging or dementia. Adults 55 and over are more severely affected by alcohol, with physiologically less tolerance, and recovery being significantly slower.

Multiple Problems

It is well-known that older persons suffer from multiple health problems and the same is observed among older homeless people. For example, a study in Boston found, on average, four major chronic illnesses in the study population (O'Connell, 1990) while a more recent survey in the same city found that close to 33% of the older adults had co-existing health and functional impairments. Hamel (2001) found in Massachusetts that 50% of the sample had two or more physical, psychological, or addictive impairments. The combination of mental health problems and excessive use of alcohol is a lethal problem for the older homeless population (Crane & Warnes, 2000).

BARRIERS AND ACCESS TO SERVICES

Several British studies have found that homeless people have difficulty accessing services (Crane, 1996). A study in the United Kingdom suggested that many older people have had no contact with a physician in several years, despite the presence of physical problems (Crane & Warnes, 2001). Reasons provided to account for this finding included: fear of illness and physicians, lack of recognition of the severity of the illness, and fear of being shunned by health professionals. Homeless people often end up accessing services in a crisis situation. Other work suggests that not having a health card (required in Canada) and reluctance of health care providers to register homeless people because they have multiple health problems (in the United Kingdom) and being difficult to track due to their transient nature, may also be barriers to accessing care (Hwang et al., 2001). In addition, a Toronto study found that, following rent, the greatest cost facing older people using food banks was medication expenses. Forty percent of these older people had difficulty paying for prescription medications each month, while 27% did not take their prescription drugs because they could not afford them (Daily Bread Food Bank, 2001).

IMPLICATIONS FOR TORONTO STUDY

The small research literature on homelessness and aging presents a fleeting snapshot of the unique characteristics of older homeless adults. In light of this research, we expected to find that elderly homeless adults in Toronto experienced difficulties finding affordable housing, that they were poor, had serious mental and physical health concerns, and were up against formidable barriers in accessing health and social services. The literature suggested that there may be differences between the long- and short-term homeless according to their paths into homelessness but did not indicate if problems were dispersed differently between the two groups, if each group had special needs, what health and social services were used by the two sub-groups, or if each group warranted different approaches to intervention. This study attempted to discern these differences in order to provide some guidance for what services were required, who needed to deliver them, and the best practices for delivering them. Our overarching goal was to further refine what we knew about older homeless adults so that services could reflect the diversity that was beginning to emerge in this sub-population.

DATA AND METHODS

The data reported here are from a larger, multi-method, descriptive study which was designed to better understand older homeless adults in Toronto and their use of housing, health, and social services (McDonald, Dergal, & Cleghorn, 2004). The study used four sources of data: secondary data analysis of hostel data originally collected by shelters for the homeless from 1987 to 2002 for the Greater Toronto Area; a survey that collected data in face-to-face interviews with 68 older homeless persons; thirty in-depth interviews with older chronic and recently homeless adults and those at risk for homelessness; and three focus groups conducted with twenty-seven staff and service providers of community-based agencies that dealt directly with older people and/or the homeless. In this paper we report on a further analysis of the cross-sectional survey data (N = 68) that compares the housing and service needs of the recent older homeless with the long-term homeless. The objective of the survey was to develop a sociodemographic profile of the older homeless, using standardized measures to augment the secondary analysis of the shelter data that, although longitudinal, did not ask extensive questions.

There are many definitions of homelessness as noted above and many ages at which adults are considered to be old. In this study we used literal homelessness as the definition to be consistent with other studies in Canada (City of Toronto, 2003; Serge & Gnaedinger, 2003). This broad definition includes people living in public places as on the street, in temporary shelters, or in locations not meant for human habitation. Literal homelessness can be chronic or short-term although these definitions vary widely. As well, literal homelessness does not take into account the hidden homeless who rarely show up at a shelter for public services (Fournier, 1998; Eberle Planning & Research, 2002). *Old* was defined as 50 years of age to be consistent with the growing consensus in the literature. Purposive sampling was utilized for the survey to ensure that older homeless people were sampled from three sectors: the hostel sector; congregate areas (e.g., sleeping outdoors, parks), and from services offered to the older people and the homeless, other than from hostels (e.g., food banks, drop-in centers, senior centers).

Sample

In order to make contact with older homeless persons in the three sectors, staff in programs and agencies who work with older people and the homeless were used as the link between the researchers and the participants. Contact was made with approximately 57 agencies that served homeless or older adults. Agency staff were asked to identify any older persons who met the sampling criteria, of 50 and over and literally homeless. Outreach programs were used to locate older persons in the congregate areas. When the agency staff identified a candidate for the interview, they asked the person if they would talk to the researchers about the study and then the researchers explained the study and asked for voluntary participation. If the participant met the criteria for the interview and decided to enter the study, a private and safe place for the interview was found that was acceptable to the respondent (a shelter, a coffee shop, a private room at the agency, etc). Signed consent was required of the participants and they were given a $20 honorarium to compensate them for their time, for which a receipt was issued. Overall, the survey questionnaire took approximately an hour to administer.

Measures

The survey questionnaire was developed through consultations with staff from agencies and shelters that serve homeless older adults. The questions and scales used in the schedules were also based on instruments used in previous studies of homelessness. Both were pre-tested and revised accordingly. The questionnaire covered many different areas: demographics, experience of homelessness, recent housing history, use of health and community services, alcohol and tobacco use, drug use, health status, nutrition, activities of daily living, social support, income, and life satisfaction. Questions were obtained from three sources. First, questions were used from a previous study done in Toronto with the homeless population (Svoboda & Kurji, 2003). For example, the questions related to alcohol and drug use were obtained from a survey already piloted and administered successfully to this group. Second, questions were used from the National Population Health Survey (NPHS), a national longitudinal and random stratified survey of the health of Canadians so that comparisons could be made to the national population. The list of health and community services, the checklist of health problems, and questions related to vision, hearing, speech, mobility, and nutrition, were similar to those in the NPHS. Finally, standardized measures were used to measure health status, orientation-memory-concentration, problem drinking, activities of daily living (ADLs), mood, and social support. These scales were chosen because they were frequently used, were easy to administer to the population in terms of length and wording, and the questions were relevant to older homeless adults.

One of the scales, the SF-12, is a generic measure of health status that has been widely used to measure health status in other studies. It consists of 12-items, and includes 1 or 2 items related to nine health concepts: physical functioning, role-physical, bodily pain, general health, energy/fatigue, social functioning, role-emotional, mental health, and change in health. There are two summary scales that are produced from the SF-12; the Physical Component Summary (PCS), and the Mental Component Summary (MCS). The scoring for both scales uses norm-based methods that have been widely used to measure health status in other studies. The Orientation-Memory-Concentration Test is a validated short version of the MMSE (Katzman, Brown, Fuld, Schechter, & Schimmel, 1983). It consists of 6 items each weighted with a different value and produces a score between 0-28, with scores over 20 considered within the normal range. The CAGE scale is a four-item, self-report test used to screen for problem drinking. Affirmative answers to each of the four items are assigned a value of 1 and a cut-off score of two or higher is considered indicative of problem drinking. Mayfield, McLeod and Hall (1974) found that a CAGE score of two or higher had a correlation of 0.89 with clinical diagnosis of alcoholism (Mayfield, McLeod & Hall, 1974).

The short form of the Geriatric Depression Scale (GDS-SF) was used to screen for depressive symptoms in participants and to evaluate the clinical severity of depression. The GDS-SF is a 15-item, self-report inventory that requires participants to respond yes or no to a series of questions regarding their mood in the previous week. The highest possible score is 15. For clinical purposes, a score greater than 5 suggests depression and warrants a follow-up interview. Probable depression is indicated by scores greater than 10 (Sheikh & Yesavage, 1986).

Data Analysis

Descriptive statistics were used for the analysis of the survey data but here our analysis compares those who became homeless prior to 50 years of age with those participants who became homeless over 50 years of age. In our bivariate analysis, we used cross tabulation for categorical data and analysis of variance for continuously measured data. The sample is small and non-representative, so tests of significance were not used.

Limitations

Although Toronto is the largest city in Canada with over 4 million people, older homeless adults were difficult to find and were quite tentative during the interviews (Crane, 1998).[2] Furthermore, the sample was non-random; it was small and localized and, by dividing it into subgroups, gender and immigrant analyses were not feasible.

FINDINGS

Sociodemographic Characteristics

The analyses of socio-demographic data indicated that there were more male older homeless adults than females, a finding consistent with the existing research on the older homeless. Of the sample, 67% were males compared to 33% females. While more males (69%) became homeless prior to age 50, females (36%) became homeless at later ages in this sample. As would be expected, the average age of the sub-group who became homeless in old age was higher–about 60 years compared to 56 years for the long-term homeless, possibly because a lifetime of living on the streets is known to affect mortality.[3] In keeping with the high immigration rates in Toronto, a larger percentage, 55% of the recent older homeless, were born outside of Canada compared to 29% of the long-term homeless. There were too few cases to identify country of origin; however, the aggregate data indicated that the majority of immigrants were from Africa and the Caribbean.

The recent older homeless were more likely to be married or widowed, a larger proportion were separated or divorced, and they were less likely to be single than the long-term homeless group. Nevertheless, the long-term homeless were more likely to be in contact with an ex-spouse; they also had more siblings and more contact with them than the recent older homeless adults. The newly homeless had more children and more grandchildren than the comparison group and they had more contact with them. These differences suggest that the recent older homeless have a different circle of family relationships than the long-term homeless that spans more than one generation.

The recent homeless had a slightly higher education than the long-term homeless and they were more likely to have been employed or recently unemployed, or at least have a closer relationship to the labor force. This fact is not reflected in their incomes, however, because the long-term homeless had greater incomes, possibly due to the fact that a larger proportion received disability and welfare benefits. The long-term homeless were more likely to receive 23% of their income from Ontario Works, a form of provincial welfare and 38% of their income from a provincial disability benefit, both of which are fairly stable benefits. Close to 42% of the recent older homeless received a Personal Needs Allowance tied to their use of shelters with a worth of about $112 per month. It is important to note that people residing in shelters are not eligible for Ontario Works benefits because it is thought that the shelter can meet their needs. None of these benefits come even close to covering the cost of housing. For example, income assistance benefits for a single individual are $520 and the average one room apartment rents for $531 in Toronto (City of

Toronto, 2003). It is worth noting that, even though more than 10% of the sample was over age 65, few were receiving Old Age Security and the Guaranteed Income Supplement, pension benefits which are income tested and which the homeless would be entitled to given their low incomes. Immigrants, however, often do not qualify for full pension benefits since the amount of the pension is based on length of residency in Canada.

Experience of Homelessness

The most obvious differences between the short-term and long-term homeless was that the recent homeless appeared to be struggling due to a lack of information about the homeless service system. Seventy percent of the adults new to homelessness had difficulties finding shelter compared to 19% of the established homeless; 57% compared to 47% did not have enough food to eat and, in the last year, they were likely to be homeless 3 weeks longer than the long-term homeless. In contrast, the long-term homeless became homeless on average at age 38, compared to age 57 for the new homeless; over half of the chronic homeless had stayed in a shelter for at least 12 months compared to 19% of the new homeless and they had been homeless a minimum of seven times since the first time they were homeless. Both the recent and long-term homeless saw homeless people as old at about 50 years of age, consistent with the research and general views of professionals in the homeless field.

The participants in the study were asked about how they became homeless in an open-ended question. The answers were complicated, usually involving a number of simultaneous issues. The main issues identified included: 18 cases of eviction; 10 situations of family breakdown for reasons of abusive and problem behaviour, widowhood and loss of a caretaker; 8 instances where the person was discharged from a hospital directly to a shelter; 10 situations related to poverty and the cold; 4 refugees who had no place to go; and several people who lost their jobs. Usually, someone would have lost their job, been evicted, or been admitted to hospital which then sent them to a shelter. The main difference for homelessness between the two groups was that the recent homeless were more likely to cite family conflicts, widowhood, and loss of a job as to why they were on the street or in a shelter. Many of these recent homeless spent a great deal more time trying to explain why they were homeless and seemed shocked at their own straitened circumstances.

The participants were asked about their current living arrangements and about the last three places they had lived. Over time, the long-term homeless reduced their time on the street with the numbers shrinking from 22 to 9%.[4] Their use of shelters over four moves went from 13% to 34%; they also moved into long-term shelters in greater numbers, the proportion growing from 3 to

20%. Their drop in the share of self-contained housing was substantial from 44% to 20%. Even though they had been in the system for some time, they still had not achieved permanent and affordable housing. Their circumstances, however, were not quite as devastating as those of the recent homeless. The share of self-contained housing of the recent homeless dropped dramatically from 45% to 7% over four moves. The housing pattern of these adults appeared to be on a fast downward slide. Their dwindling share of room and board occupancy went from 23% to 7%, a form of *at-risk-housing*, while their use of emergency shelters rose from 10 to 52%. Their presence on the street over four moves stayed the same at about 13% in contrast to the reduced percentage of long-term adults remaining on the streets. The recent homeless also were not as likely to be in long-term shelters as the long-term older homeless were.

Health

As Table 1 indicates, the SF-12 physical score was very low for both the recent and long-term homeless with the recent homeless having a slightly lower score of 33.68 compared to 35.83 for the chronic homeless. The average score of the two groups, 35.01, was much lower than the score of 46.12 for the general U.S. population of the same age.[5] Indeed, the general score for the older homeless was lower than the norm of 38.68 for people over age 75 in the U.S. general population. Although the number of cases is small, the scaled norms suggest that according to physical health indicators, the homeless were physically older than their chronological age. The score for mental health of 45.09 for the recent homeless was slightly lower than the 47.74 score for the life long homeless, and both were lower for the norms for the general U.S. population for the age groups 55 to 64, (50.57) and for those 75 plus (50.06). In Canada 28% of those 65 and older report a memory problem compared to 74% of the long-term homeless and 72% of the recent homeless (Lindsay, 1999).

Table 1 provides a list of the top 12 health problems suffered by both sub-groups. Like many earlier localized studies, the top five health problems for the long-term homeless included memory issues, dental problems, vision problems, alcohol concerns, and back problems. In comparison, the top five problems for the recent homeless were arthritis and depression followed by vision, alcohol and back problems. Therefore, the main health problems differed substantially between the two sub-groups: memory and dental issues were problems for the long-term homeless compared to arthritis and depression for the recent homeless. In the Canadian population 65 and over in 1996, the most reported chronic illnesses were arthritis, high blood pressure, heart disease and diabetes (Lindsay, 1999).[6] Overall, a larger proportion of the homeless suffered from some of these diseases. Arthritis, endured by 32.2% of the Canadian

TABLE 1. Health Problems of Homelessness, Past Six Months 2004*

Problems	Percentages		
	Homeless before 50	Homeless after 50	Total
SF-12 Physical Score			
Mean	35.83 (13)	33.68 (8)	35.01 (21)
Standard deviation	3.72	4.25	3.98
SF-12 Mental Score			
Mean	47.74 (13)	45.09 (8)	46.73
Standard Deviation	5.73	9.13	7.11
Memory and Orientation			
Normal	26 (6)	28 (5)	27 (11)
Problems	74 (17)	72 (13)	73 (30)
Teeth and Gums			
Yes	69 (24)	36 (11)	53 (35)
No	31 (4)	65 (20)	47 (31)
Vision/Needs Glasses			
Yes	58 (11)	42 (8)	50 (19)
No	42 (8)	58 (11)	50 (19)
Alcohol Problems (CAGE)			
Yes	58 (11)	42 (8)	50 (19)
No	42 (8)	58 (11)	50 (19)
Back Problems (not arthritis)			
Yes	54 (19)	42 (13)	49 (32)
No	46 (16)	58 (18)	52 (34)
Arthritis/Rheumatism			
Yes	51 (18)	61 (19)	56 (37)
No	49 (17)	39 (12)	44 (29)
Nerves/Anxiety			
Yes	37 (13)	39 (12)	38 (25)
No	63 (22)	61 (19)	62 (41)
Depression			
Possible Depression	37 (10)	50 (12)	43 (22)
Not Depressed	63 (17)	50 (12)	57 (29)
Bronchitis			
Yes	26 (9)	23 (7)	24 (16)
No	74 (26)	77 (24)	76 (50)
Blood Pressure			
Yes	24 (8)	42 (13)	32 (21)
No	77 (26)	58 (18)	68 (44)
Diarrhea			
Yes	17 (6)	16 (5)	17 (11)
No	83 (29)	84 (26)	83 (55)
Injuries			
Yes	17 (6)	27 (7)	20 (13)
No	83 (29)	77 (24)	80 (53)

* Number of cases in brackets

elderly, affected 56% of all the homeless and was seriously over-represented amongst the recent homeless. Sixty-one percent reported that a nurse or doctor had diagnosed this problem at some time. Although 15.4% of the Canadian population report back problems, 49% of the homeless noted this problem, especially the long-term homeless. More homeless people reported high blood pressure than the general population. Approximately 42% of the recent homeless reported this problem compared to 28% for the population 65 and over.

Dental problems, anxiety, diarrhea, and depression are diseases the general population is less likely to note (Lindsay, 1999). The differences between the two sub-groups of older homeless persons appeared to be related to the street *life-style* of the homeless adults who managed to age in place, with the concomitant problems of higher levels of memory deficits, alcoholism, diarrhea, and bronchitis. The afflictions of the short-term homeless who had arthritis, blood pressure concerns, probable depression, and anxiety and who had been injured (over 25%) appeared to be responses to a very difficult environment for which they were not prepared. Given these health concerns, only a small proportion of each sub-group received treatment or used the appropriate services.

Table 2 indicates that the long-term homeless clearly relied on emergency services of all types from use of hospital emergency rooms (51% compared to 36% of the recent homeless) to street outreach (23% compared to no utilization). The difference in the use of street outreach services shows how unacquainted the recent homeless were with services for the homeless since more of them were on the street than the long-term elderly. The recent homeless tended to use health services in the long and short term shelters where they resided and, although they were less likely to have an alcohol problem, they availed themselves of addiction services. It is interesting to note that none of them used ethno-specific services although they were more likely to have been born outside of Canada. Although 89% of Canadian adults age 65 and over saw their general practitioner at least once a year (Lindsay, 1999), in this sample, only 39% of recent homeless and 47% of the long-term homeless visited a private doctor's office in the last six months. Only 19% of the recent homeless compared to 18% of the chronic homeless visited walk-in clinics, although 81% of the recent homeless said they had health cards compared to 77% of the chronic homeless.

An examination of the reported barriers to the use of health care in a country with universal health care is telling. Overall, larger percentages of the recent homeless identified barriers to health care than did the long-term homeless. Not having a health card definitely prevented the recent homeless (40%) in contrast with the long-term homeless (20%) from using services, although no one would ever be refused help. Over seventy-one percent of the

TABLE 2. Use of Medical Services (Last 6 Months) Homelessness 2004*

Problems	Percentages		
	Homeless before 50	Homeless after 50	Total
Has Health Card			
Yes	77 (27)	81 (25)	79 (52)
No	23 (8)	19 (6)	21 (14)
Hospital Admittance			
Yes	40 (14)	29 (9)	35 (23)
No	60 (21)	61 (22)	65 (43)
Hospital Emergency Room			
Yes	51 (18)	36 (11)	44 (29)
No	49 (17)	65 (20)	56 (37)
Prescribed Medications			
Yes	74 (26)	74 (23)	74 (49)
No	26 (9)	26 (8)	26 (17)
Shelter Health Services			
Yes	14 (5)	29 (9)	21 (14)
No	86 (30)	71 (22)	79 (52)
Drop-in Centre			
Yes	37 (13)	.....	21 (14)
No	63 (22)	97 (30)	79 (52)
Walk-in Clinic			
Yes	18 (6)	19 (6)	19 (12)
No	82 (27)	81 (25)	81 (52)
Private Doctor			
Yes	47 (16)	39 (12)	43 (28)
No	53 (18)	61 (19)	57 (37)
Addiction Treatment Centre			
Yes	....	16 (5)	12 (8)
No	91 (31)	84 (26)	88 (57)
Emergency Response Team			
Yes	26 (9)	.....	19 (12)
No	74 (26)	90 (26)	81 (52)
Community Health Centre			
Yes	32 (11)	....	19 (12)
No	68 (23)	98 (30)	82 (53)
Street Outreach			
Yes	23 (9)	....	15 (10)
No	77 (27)	94 (29)	85 (56)

* Number of cases in brackets
… Following Statistics Canada guidelines, estimates cannot be reported because of insufficient cases.

recent homeless felt that the waiting time was too long for service, almost 60% felt that they could not afford the cost or the cost of a prescription service (some services are not covered by health care), 43% couldn't get to the service because they did not have a means of transportation, 43% had little hope that the service would be adequate, 14% were afraid of doctors, and 27% felt that they would be discriminated against by service providers.

In contrast, 64% of long-term homeless noted that the service they required was not available at the time they required it and 29% indicated that they didn't bother with the service, reasons perhaps consistent with the immediacy of their transient life style.

As was the case with health services, the recent homeless did not use community services as extensively as the long-term homeless, as illustrated in Table 3. In fact, there were many services they did not use at all, such as food banks, mental health services, legal services, services for older adults, and employment services, although they were older and had a stronger link to the labor force. The recent homeless appeared to be focused on the obvious–53% used the housing help services to try and find a place to live. The long-term homeless were more likely to use the services found in the homeless sector, no one used mental health services which were urgently needed, and only 17% used services designed for older persons. The long-term homeless apparently did not give up on searching for housing since 40% still used housing help services. The message here is that the recent homeless did not appear to use the services that were available to them for whatever reasons–newness to homelessness, lack of information from service providers, no access, the limitations of the shelter system where they tended to reside, or the inappropriateness of services. Although they were older they never used services especially designed for older people. The long-term homeless, while still trying to house themselves after being on the streets for close to twenty years, were depending on short-term and temporary services like drop-in centers for meals and spending time in public places like the library and religious institutions.

In terms of the professional contact, long-term homeless adults were more likely to see, in order of importance: pharmacists (45%), social workers (34%), the police (19%), psychiatrists (11%), and mental health nurses (9%). The recent homeless were more likely to visit an eye specialist (38%), a dentist (24%), and a physiotherapist (10%). Equal proportions of both groups visited a podiatrist (22%) and an occupational therapist (2%). The proportions that saw professionals were not nearly large enough to match the degree of reported health problems. For example, about 17% of the long-term homeless and 36% of the new homeless saw an eye specialist when 58% of the long-term and 42% of the recent homeless reported vision problems.

TABLE 3. Use of Community Services (Last 6 Months) Homelessness 2004*

Problems	Percentages		
	Homeless before 50	Homeless after 50	Total
Drop-in Centre to Socialize			
Yes	74 (26)	53 (16)	42 (42)
No	26 (9)	47 (14)	35 (23)
Drop-in Centre for Meals			
Yes	74 (26)	50 (15)	63 (41)
No	26 (9)	50 (15)	37 (24)
Foodbank Meal Program			
Yes	40 (14)	0 (0)	22 (14)
No	60 (21)	100 (30)	79 (51)
Counselling Services			
Yes	23 (8)	23 (7)	23 (15)
No	77 (27)	77 (23)	77 (50)
Mental Health Service			
Yes	.....	.....	8 (5)
No	87 (31)	97 (29)	92 (60)
Church, Mosque or Temple			
Yes	49 (17)	33 (10)	42 (27)
No	51 (18)	67 (20)	59 (38)
Legal Service			
Yes	26 (9)	....	20 (13)
No	74 (26)	87 (26)	80 (52)
Housing Help Service			
Yes	40 (14)	53 (16)	46 (30)
No	60 (21)	47 (14)	54 (35)
Ethno-Specific Service			
Yes	. . .	. . .	94 (61)
No	. . .	. . .	6 (4)
Services for Older Adults			
Yes	17 (6)	. . .*	14 (9)
No	83 (29)	90 (27)	86 (56)
Library			
Yes	57 (20)	33 (10)	46 (30)
No	43 (15)	67 (20)	54 (35)
Gerontological Services			
Yes	17 (6)	....	14 (9)
No	83 (29)	90 (27)	86 (56)
Employment Service			
Yes	....	....	8 (5)
No	88 (30)	97 (29)	92 (59)

* Number of cases in brackets
... Following Statistics Canada guidelines, estimates cannot be reported because of insufficient cases.

Similarly, while arthritis was a serious problem for both groups, only a small proportion of each group saw physiotherapy or occupational therapists. If 50% of the recent homeless and 37% of the chronic homeless suffered from depression, and only 8% (recent) and 11% (long-term) saw a psychiatrist, there are genuine problems in securing treatment. In light of the fact that at least three quarters of each group experienced memory and cognition problems, it is disquieting that only 9% of the long-term homeless and none of the recent homeless saw a mental health nurse.

Service providers were identified as the foundation of social life for the long-term homeless (43%) while friends were identified as the preferred social supports for the short-term homeless (48%). The seasoned street adults preferred to talk with service providers and say they actually talked with them. In contrast, the recent homeless said they preferred to talk with their friends but ended up spending equal time talking with service providers in the homeless sector.

In summary, the data suggest that the long-term homeless have different needs, see different service providers, and use different services compared to the recent older homeless. There is even some question as to whether the services delivered match the needs of either group, given the under utilization of gerontological services and the reliance on short-term solutions to protracted problems. The two sub-groups experienced different obstacles to service delivery that indicated a lack of knowledge and naiveté on the part of the recent homeless and the adaptation of the long-term homeless to the homeless milieu (Cohen, 1999; Gounis & Susser, 1990; Vance, 1994).

IMPLICATIONS FOR SOCIAL WORK

This study moves our knowledge one step further by identifying some of the differences between the long-term and recently older homeless in a localized study in Toronto. The data are quite consistent with the existing studies but provide a little more detail about the different types of older homeless people. The study indicated that more women than men became homeless at later ages, that the recent homeless were at least four years older than the long-term homeless and were closer to their sixties than fifties. Over half of the recent homeless were immigrants to Canada and were probably from the Caribbean and Africa. The short-term homeless suffered more family breakdowns, had less contact with ex-spouses and siblings but did have more contact with children and grandchildren. They had a stronger relationship to the work force but their incomes were lower than the long-term elderly because they were less likely to be receiving permanent benefits. They experienced more trouble finding food and shelter; their most recent episode of homelessness was longer than the long-term homeless and over half lived in an emergency shelter.

While the long-term homeless had reduced their presence on the street, a large proportion still resided in emergency shelters. Nonetheless, some had managed to move on to long-term shelters or back to a tenuous, but self-contained housing. The recent older homeless remained on the street or in emergency shelters over their last four moves. Both groups experienced very poor physical health compared to the general population but their illnesses were different. The recent homeless were afflicted with arthritis and depression, while the long-term homeless were more likely to experience dental and vision problems. The long-term homeless generally experienced more problems with mental health including memory and cognition problems and alcohol addiction. The short-term homeless barely used any social services at all and more of them identified barriers to health care service. The long-term homeless were more likely to rely on emergency health services and made more use of crisis type social services. The recent homeless were most intent on using services to help them find a place to live, and after many years on the street, even the long-term homeless were still trying to find housing. The long-term homeless were more likely to see pharmacy and social work professionals, while the recent homeless had less contact with professionals overall, except for eye specialists and dentists, professionals not exactly concerned with homelessness. In both sub-groups, the numbers that saw professionals were not nearly large enough to match the degree of reported health problems.

The differences highlighted by this analysis raise a number of issues for social work practitioners. It seems fairly clear that the housing issues vary between the two sub-groups and require different approaches. Certainly, affordable housing is needed to address homelessness in general, but we would argue that interventions to find housing for the recent older homeless should be swift and immediate and would be one of the first priorities of intervention in order to prevent entrenchment in street life (Cohen, 1999). The argument cannot be made that these older people consider the emergency shelter their permanent home and should not be moved (Gibeau, 2001). Supportive housing, where *maintenance is progress* seemed indicated, a principle in the care of older adults that gerontological social workers have always promoted. In short, moving the recently older homeless quickly to the gerontological sector for help would likely be more beneficial to the older person. No matter what the setting, all social workers need be on the lookout for recently homeless older adults, especially in general hospital settings. At minimum, criteria indicating homelessness should be covered in social work assessments of older adults (Gibeau, 2001). The data strongly indicated that to treat these adults as chronically homeless, when they are not, is to do them a disservice.

Hecht and Coyle (2001) make a disturbing observation when they argue that the discourse on the older homeless problem, its solutions and practices, often contradicts what gerontologists know about the housing needs of older people. In particular, they flag the whole issue of crisis intervention and the focus on independence and self-sufficiency, models more befitting the young homeless. The data here underscore the interminable round of crises experienced by the long-term homeless and their need for permanent solutions that remove them from the merry-go-round of emergency departments, drop-ins, and food banks. While some of these adults may prefer street life, the fact that 40% were still using housing help services is compelling. Long-term and joint planning between the homeless and gerontology service sectors that nurtures the older person over the long haul, instead of providing a patchwork of uncoordinated and temporary services, seems indicated. Permanently supported living arrangements in which the level of support increases as need increases is not new to gerontology and could be made available for chronic older homeless persons. The whole shelter system, including long term shelters, as currently organized with their focus on short-term assistance, could actually be seen as prolonging the homeless situation of older adults who became homeless before the age fifty.

Finally, the dissonance between self-identified needs and services in this survey should be enough to make social work take stock since they are the main service professionals seen by the older homeless. The needs for health care and social services are different for the two groups, but it appears that the needs of neither sub-group are met. The magnitudes of the health and social problems far outstrip the services rendered. The very limited provision of basic physical and mental health care, especially needed for the long-term homeless, is hard to comprehend in a country with universal health care. We can only conclude that both sub-groups require extraordinary efforts to help them access the applicable services. The need for advocacy, more and thorough follow-up, and case management is necessary for the long-term homeless. The recent homeless require knowledge and information about the services available to them. These services should be rendered in a supportive and non-judgmental atmosphere that is culturally and linguistically sensitive. It is recognized that the decline in affordable housing, the slashing of welfare budgets, and the closure of hospitals and clinics is the context within which the baby boomers are aging. There is no reason, however, why the two existing services sectors could not pool their resources in the service of the older homeless while the bigger issues are fought on the policy front.

This study is not without flaws that are inherent to studies of the homeless. In future, larger samples from equivalent-sized cities and samples from smaller cities would help clarify the needs of the two subgroups of older adults. Larger samples would also facilitate a gender analysis and an analysis of the service needs of new immigrants for whom we have virtually no reliable information. Lastly, the few unique models for delivery of health and social services for older adults need to be evaluated.

NOTES

1. The older homeless, however, are believed to constitute a diminishing proportion of the total homeless population (Burt, 1992; Cohen, 1999; Crane & Warnes, 2001). The lower percentage of homelessness amongst the elderly has been attributed to the availability of entitlements like social security, and to 'survival effects,' meaning that homeless adults may not survive to age sixty-five (Cohen, 1999).

2. The social housing waiting list in Toronto is 71,000 as of 2003. In 2002, 31,985 persons stayed in shelters and 4,779 were children (City of Toronto, 2003).

3. The age range in the sample was from 50 to over 80 years. Forty-two percent were 50 to 55; 16% 56 to 59; 22% 60 to 65; 4%, 66 to 69; 6% 70 to 75; 6% 76 plus and 4% missing.

4. For the purposes of this study, emergency shelter use was defined as 3 months or less continuous residence, and long-term shelter use was defined as over 3 months continuous residence.

5. SF-12 scores for the general Canadian population are not available.

6. More recent data has not been released by Statistics Canada.

REFERENCES

Abdul-Hamid, W. (1997). The elderly homeless men in Bloomsbury hostels: Their needs for services. *International Journal of Geriatric Psychiatry, 12,* 724-727.

Acorn, S. (1993). Mental and physical health of homeless persons who use emergency shelters in Vancouver. *Hospital and Community Psychiatry, 44*(9), 854-857.

Applewhite, S. L. (1997). Homeless Veterans: Perspectives on Social Service Use. *Social Work, 42*(1), 19-30.

Ashe, J., Brandon, J., Contogouris, M., & Swanson, M. (1996). *The San Francisco Homeless Death Review: Revised Preliminary Report 1996.* San Francisco: San Francisco Department of Public Health.

Auslander, L. A., & Jeste, D. V. (2002). Perceptions of problems and needs for service among middle-aged and elderly outpatients with schizophrenia and related psychotic disorders. *Community Mental Health Journal, 38*(5), 391-402.

Avramov, D. (1995). *Homelessness in the European Union: Social and legal context of housing exclusion in the 1990s.* Fourth Research Report of the European Observatory on Homelessness. Brussels, Belgium: European Federation of National Organizations Working with the Homeless.

Barrow, S. M., Hermann, D. B., Cordova, P., & Struening, E. L. (1999). Mortality among homeless shelter residents in New York City. *American Journal of Public Health, 89*(4), 529-534.

Bottomley, J. M., Bissonette, A., & Snekvik, V. C. (2001). The lives of homeless older adults: Please tell them who I am. *Topics in Geriatric Rehabilitation, 16*(4), 50-65.

Boucher, L. (1995). Substance abuse. In D. Wiatt Rich, T. Rich & L. Mullins (Eds.), *Old and homeless–double jeopardy.* Westport: Auburn House.

British Colombia Ministry of Social Development and Economic Security, a. B. H. M. C. (2001). *Homelessness–causes and effects: A review of the literature.*

Bruckner, J. (2001). Walking a mile in their shoes. *Topics in Geriatric Rehabilitation, 16*(4), 15-27.

Buhrich, N., Hodder, T., & Teesson, M. (2000). Prevalence of cognitive impairment among homeless people in inner Sydney. *Psychiatric Services, 51*(4), 520-509.

Burnette, D., Morrow-Howell, N., & Chen, L. (2003). Setting priorities for gerontological social work: A national Delphi study. *The Gerontologist, 43*(6), 828-839.

Burt, M. R. (1992). *Over the edge: The growth of homelessness in the 1980s.* New York: Russell Sage Foundation.

City of Toronto (2003). *The Toronto Report Card on Housing and Homelessness.* Toronto.

Cohen, C. I., Tresi, J., Holmes, D., & Roth, E. (1988). Survival strategies of older homeless men. *The Gerontologist, 28*(1), 58-65.

Cohen, C. I., & Sokolovsky, J. (1989). *Old men of the Bowery: Strategies for survival among the homeless.* New York: Guilford.

Cohen, C. I., Onserud, H., & Monaco, C. (1992). Project rescue: Serving the homeless and marginally housed elderly. *The Gerontologist, 32*(4), 466-471.

Cohen, C. I., & Crane, M. (1996). Old and homeless in London and New York City: A cross-national comparison. In D. Bhurga (Ed.), *Homelessness and Mental Health* (pp. 150-169). London: Cambridge University Press.

Cohen, C. I., Ramirez, M., Teresi, J., Gallagher, M., & Sokolovsky, J. (1997). Predictors of becoming redomiciled among older homeless women. *The Gerontologist, 37*(1), 67-74.

Cohen, C. I. (1999). Aging and homelessness. *The Gerontologist, 39*(1), 5-14.

Council of Social Work Education (2001). *A blueprint for the new millennium.* Alexandria VA: CSWE.

Crane, M. (1994). The mental health problems of elderly people living on London's streets. *International Journal of Geriatric Psychiatry, 9,* 87-95.

Crane, M. (1996). The situation of older homeless people. *Reviews in Clinical Gerontology, 6,* 389-398.

Crane, M. (1998). The associations between mental illness and homelessness among older people: An exploratory study. *Aging & Mental Health, 2*(3), 171-180.

Crane, M., & Warnes, A. M. (2000). *Lessons from Lancefield Street: Tackling the needs of older homeless people.* London: National Homeless Alliance.

Crane, M., & Warnes, A. M. (2001). Primary health care services for single people: Defects and opportunities. *Family Practice–An International Journal, 18*(3), 272-276.

Daily Bread Food Bank. (2001). *Aging with Dignity?: How governments create insecurity for low-income seniors.* Toronto.

DeMallie, D., North, C., & Smith, E. (1997). Psychiatric disorders among the homeless: A comparison of older and younger groups. *The Gerontologist, 37*(1), 61-66.

Doolin, J. (1986). Planning for the social needs of the homeless elderly. *The Gerontologist, 26*(3), 229-231.

Eberle Planning and Research. (2002). *Research project on homelessness in greater Vancouver: Profile of homeless and at-risk people in greater Vancouver.* Vancouver: The Greater Vancouver Regional District.

Fischer, P. J., & Breakey, W. R. (1991). The epidemiology of alcohol, drug, and mental disorders among homeless persons. *American Psychologist, 46,* 1115-1128.

Fisher, N., Turner, S. W., Pugh, R., & Taylor, C. (1994). Estimating numbers of homeless and homeless mentally ill people in north east Westminster by using capture-recapture analysis. *BMJ, 308,* 27-30.

Fournier, L. (1998). *Denombrement de la clientele itinerante dans les entres d'hebegement, les soupes populaires et les centres de jour des villes de Montreal et de Quebec 1996-1997:* Sante Quebec.

Gelberg, L., Linn, L. S., & Mayer-Oakes, S. A. (1990). Differences in health status between older and younger homeless adults. *JAGS, 38,* 1220-1229.

Gibeau, J. L. (2001). Home free: An evolving journey in eradicating elder homelessness. *Topics in Geriatric Rehabilitation, 17*(1), 22-52.

Gounis, K., & Susser, E. (1990). Shelterization and its implications for mental health services. In N. L. Cohen (Ed.), *Psychiatry takes to the street* (pp. 231-255). New York: Guilford.

Greve, J. (1991). *Homelessness in Britain.* York, England: Rowntree Foundation.

Hallebone, E. (1997). Homelessness and marginality in Australia: Young and old people excluded from independence. In M. Huth & T. Wright (Eds.), *International critical perspectives on homelessness* (pp. 69-103). Westport, CT: Praeger.

Hamel, P. (2001). Interdisciplinary perspectives, service learning and advocacy: A non-traditional approach to geriatric rehabilitation. *Topics in Geriatric Rehabilitation 17*(1), 53-70.

Hecht, L., & Coyle, B. (2001). Elderly homeless: A comparison of older and younger adult emergency shelter seekers. *American Behavioural Scientist, 45*(1), 66-79.

Hibbs, J. R., Benne, L., Klugman, L., Spencer, R., Macchia, I., Mellinger, A. K. et al. (1994). Mortality in a cohort of homeless adults in Philadelphia. *The New England Journal of Medicine, 331*(5), 304-309.

Hwang, S. W., Orav, E. J., O'Connell, J. J., Lebow, J. M., & Brennan, T. A. (1997). Causes of death in homeless adults in Boston. *Annals of Internal Medicine, 126*(8), 625-628.

Hwang, S. W. (2000). Mortality among men using homeless shelters in Toronto, Ontario. *JAMA, 283*(16), 2152-2157.

Hwang, S. W., O'Connell, J. J., Lebow, J. M., Bierer, M. F., Orav, E. J., & Brennan, T. A. (2001). Health care utilization among homeless adults prior to death. *Journal of Health Care for the Poor and Underserved, 12*(1), 50-59.

Katzman, R., Brown, T., Fuld, P., Schechter, R., & Schimmel, H. (1983). Validation of a short Orientation-Memory-Concentration Test of cognitive impairment. *American Journal of Psychiatry, 140,* 734-739.

Keigher, S. M., & Greenblatt, S. (1992). Housing emergencies and the etiology of homelessness among the urban elderly. *The Gerontologist, 32*(4), 457-465.

Kershaw, A., Singleton, N., & Meltzer, H. (2000). *Survey of the health and well-being of homeless people in Glasgow.* Summary Report, Office for National Statistics, London.

Killion, C. M. (2000). Extending the extended family for homeless and marginally housed African American women. *Public Health Nursing, 17*(5), 346-354.

Kisor, A. J., & Kendal-Wilson, L. (2002). Older homeless women: Reframing the stereotype of the bag lady. *AFFILIA, 17*(3), 354-370.

Kramer, J., & Barker, J. C. (1996). Homelessness among older American Indians, Los Angeles, 1987-1989. *Human Organization, 55*(4), 396-408.

Kushner, C. (1998). Better access, better care: A research paper on health services and homelessness in Toronto. *Report to the Mayor's Homelessness Action Task Force, Taking Responsibility for Homelessness,* Background papers, Vol 1.

Kutza, E. A., & Keigher, S. M. (1991). The elderly "new homeless": An emerging population at risk. *Social Work, 36*(4), 288-293.

Ladner, S. (1992). The elderly homeless. In M. J. Robertson & M. Greenblatt (Eds.), *Homelessness: A national perspective.* New York: Plenum Press.

Lindsay, C. (1999). A portrait of seniors in Canada. Statistics Canada: Housing, Family and Social Statistics Division, Ottawa. Catalogue no. 89-519-XPE.

Mayfield, D., McLeod, G., & Hall, P. (1974). The CAGE questionnaire: Validation of a new alcoholism instrument. *American Journal of Psychiatry, 131,* 1121-1123.

McDonald, L. Dergal, J., & Cleghorn, L. (2004). *Homeless Older Adults Research Project.* Final Report. Toronto.

Morbey, H., Pannell, J., & Means, R. (2003). Surviving at the margins: Older homeless people accessing housing and support. *Housing, Care and Support, 6*(1), 8-13.

North, C. S., & Smith, E. M. (1993). A systematic study of mental health services utilization by homeless men and women. *Social Psychiatry and Psychiatric Epidemiology, 28,* 77-83.

O'Connell, J. J. (1990). Caring for the homeless elderly. *Pride Institute Journal of Long-Term Home Health Care, 9*(1), 20-25.

O'Connell, J. J., Summerfield, J., & Kellogg, F. R. (1990). The homeless elderly. In P. W. Brickner, L. K. Scharer, B. A. Connan, M. Savarese, & B. C. Scanlan (Eds.). *Under the safety net: The health and social welfare of the homeless in the United States.* New York: W. W. Norton and Company.

O'Reilly-Fleming, T. (1993). *Down and out in Canada: Homeless Canadians.* Toronto: Canadian Scholars Press.

Piliavin, I., Wright, B., Mare, R., & Westerfelt, A. (1996). Exits from and returns to homelessness. *Social Service Review, 70*(1), 33-57.

Robertson, M. J., & Greenblatt, M. (1992). *Homelessness: A National Perspective.* New York: Plenum.

Rosenheck, R., & Seibyl, C. L. (1998). Homelessness: Health service use and related costs. *Medical Care, 36*(8), 1256-1264.

Rosenheck, R., Bassuk, E., & Salomon, A. (1999). Special populations of homeless Americans. In L. Fosburg & D. Dennis (Eds.), *Practical lessons: The 1998 national symposium on homeless research* (chap. 3). Prepared for US Department of Housing and Urban Development, and Department of Health and Human Services.

Rossi, P. H. (1989). *Down and out in America: The origins of homelessness.* Chicago: University of Chicago Press.

Roth, D., Tomey, B. G., & First, R. J. (1992). Gender, racial, and age variations among homeless persons. In M. J. Robertson & M. Greenblatt (Eds.), *Homelessness: A national perspective.* New York: Plenum Press.

Serge, L., & Gnaedinger, N. (2003). *Housing options for elderly or chronically ill shelter users: Final report* (No. CMHC C.R. File No. 6530-62). Ottawa: Research Division: Canadian Mortgage and Housing Corporation.

Sheikh, J. I., & Yesavage, J. A. (1986). Geriatric Depression Scale (GDS): Recent evidence and development of a shorter version. *Clinical Gerontologist, 5*(1&2), 165-173.

Springer, J., Mars, J., & Dennison, M. (1998). *A profile of the Toronto homeless population* (No. Prepared for the Mayor's Homelessness Action Task Force). Toronto: City of Toronto.

Statistics Canada. (2002). *2001 Census: Collective Dwellings* (No. 96F0030XIE2001004). Ottawa: Statistics Canada.

Stergiopoulos, V., & Herrmann, N. (2003). Old and homeless: A review and survey of older adults who use shelters in an urban setting. *Canadian Journal of Psychiatry, 48*(6), 374-380.

Svoboda, T., & Kurji, R. (2003). St. Michael's Hospital and Seaton House Men's Homeless Shelter Continuum of Care/Integration Initiative. *Journal of Urban Health, 80*(S2): ii76.

Tully, C. T., & Jacobson, S. (1994). The homeless elderly: America's forgotten population. *Journal of Gerontological Social Work, 22*(3/4), 61-80.

Vance, D. (1994). Barriers to use of services by older adults. *Psychological Reports, 75*, 1377-1378.

Vermette, G. (1994). L'itérance Chez les personnes Âgée, Régie régionale de le santéet des services sociaux de Montréal-Centre, Montréal.

Wolch, J., Dear, M., & Akita, A. (1988). Explaining homelessness. *Journal of American Planning Association, 54*, 443-453.

Wong, I., Culhane, D., & Kuhn, R. (1997). Predictors of exit and reentry among family shelter users in New York City. *Social Services Review, 71*(3), 441-462.

Wright, J. D., Rubin, B. A., & Devine, J. A. (1998). *Beside the golden door: Policy, politics and the homeless.* NY: Aldine de Gruyter.

doi:10.1300/J083v49n01_02

Housing Disparities, Caregiving, and Their Impact for Older Puerto Ricans

Blanca M. Ramos, PhD, CSW

SUMMARY. The needs of older persons in historically oppressed racial and ethnic populations remain "invisible" in the public arena (Wallace & Villa, 1999). Understanding the ethnocultural factors that shape their housing needs is essential to effective, equitable policy formation and program planning. This article examines the impact of housing disparities, health status, and cultural patterns of caregiving in relation to older Puerto Ricans on the U.S. mainland. Following a literature review of the socio-economic, living arrangement, and cultural profiles of older Puerto Ricans, policy recommendations to advance adequate housing options for this population are provided. The article concludes with a discussion of Section 202 housing policies and how they can be adapted to the current and emerging population of older Puerto Ricans. doi:10.1300/J083v49 n01_03 *[Article copies available for a fee from The Haworth Document Delivery Service: 1-800-HAWORTH. E-mail address: <docdelivery@haworthpress.com> Website: <http://www.HaworthPress.com> © 2007 by The Haworth Press, Inc. All rights reserved.]*

KEYWORDS. Housing, caregiving, older Puerto Ricans

[Haworth co-indexing entry note]: "Housing Disparities, Caregiving, and Their Impact for Older Puerto Ricans." Ramos, Blanca M. Co-published simultaneously in *Journal of Gerontological Social Work* (The Haworth Press, Inc.) Vol. 49, No. 1/2, 2007, pp. 47-64; and: *Housing for the Elderly: Policy and Practice Issues* (ed: Philip McCallion) The Haworth Press, Inc., 2007, pp. 47-64. Single or multiple copies of this article are available for a fee from The Haworth Document Delivery Service [1-800-HAWORTH, 9:00 a.m. - 5:00 p.m. (EST). E-mail address: docdelivery@haworthpress.com].

Available online at http://jgsw.haworthpress.com
© 2007 by The Haworth Press, Inc. All rights reserved.
doi:10.1300/J083v49n01_03

INTRODUCTION

As attention is focused on the housing needs of older adults, it is essential to keep in mind that living arrangements are intrinsically linked to cultural patterns of care. Further, in U.S. society, ethnic group membership, which ascribes minority status to certain groups, can inexorably influence an elder's housing and caregiving options. Ethnicity designates people on the basis of nation of origin, heritage, and cultural distinctiveness, and places elders in stratified positions where opportunities and privileges are unequally distributed (Pearlin, Mullan, Semple, & Skall, 1990). For older ethnic minority persons, this unequal distribution and differential treatment signify social disadvantage, disempowerment, and collective discrimination (Aguirre & Turner, 1995). For example, Latinos continue to lag significantly behind Whites in housing wealth as evidenced by their disadvantage in homeownership and substandard housing conditions (Flippen, 2001). This disparity invariably results in multiple housing needs, which are closely linked to few caregiving alternatives. Effective, equitable policies and programs must take into account the ethnocultural factors that shape the housing needs and attendant caregiving imperatives of elders in historically neglected minority groups.

This article examines the housing plight of older Puerto Ricans as it relates to changes in patterns of living arrangements and caregiving. Puerto Ricans are one of the most socially and economically disadvantaged populations of the Latino ethnic minority group. Although Latinos share language and cultural traits such as familism, their ethnocultural realities are qualitatively distinct due primarily to subgroup differences in sociopolitical history, racial, and ancestral backgrounds, and the way they come into contact with mainstream society (Ramos, 1997). For example, a unique characteristic of the Puerto Rican population is its U.S. citizenship status, which is granted at birth whether born on the mainland or the Island. An easy access to the mainland without immigration restrictions and wages and employment conditions in both Puerto Rico and the U.S. partly explain their back-and-forth migration pattern (Rivera-Batiz & Santiago, 1994). This ability to sojourn on the Island may contribute to a continuous reaffirmation of mainland Puerto Ricans' cultural roots. For some older adults over time, uprooting and its accompanying disruptions in family life might have contributed to a qualitatively distinct aging experience. Given Latinos' substantial within-group diversity, including documented differences in patterns of living arrangements (De Vos & Arias, 2003), it is important to examine separately the specific dynamics of this subpopulation.

The article first describes the housing situation and health status of older Puerto Ricans as these interact with ethnocultural factors. Next, the relevance of the Section 202 Supportive Housing for the Elderly Program is discussed.

Section 202 is the primary federally-funded program focused on constructing subsidized rental housing for older persons and is intended to promote their independence with shelter and supportive services. Recommendations will be offered for strengthening Section 202 to more effectively meet the housing needs of older Puerto Ricans so they can *age in place*.

PUERTO RICAN OLDER ADULTS IN THE U.S. MAINLAND: HOUSING AND HEALTH DISPARITIES

The current cohort of older Puerto Ricans includes predominantly persons who have resided on the mainland since the late 1940s as well as those who have come more recently accompanying younger relatives or to reunite with previously arrived children (Delgado & Tennstedt, 1997). Among Puerto Ricans residing in the Continental U.S., most (59.7%) were born on the mainland (U.S. Census, 2001).

Despite recent inroads among some of its members, as a group, Puerto Ricans have not fared well, and their aging population remains far removed from the American dream of upward mobility, economic opportunity, and freedom of choice (Parrillo, 2000). As an ethnic minority, many older adults have experienced life-long oppression and still face the consequences of having lived during times when overt racism and discrimination were more openly practiced (Ramos, Jones, & Toseland, 2005). Further, those with an African heritage are also vulnerable to the same harmful skin-color prejudices confronting most black Americans (Aguirre & Turner, 1995). Society's ageist attitudes and behaviors add to a lifetime of oppressive conditions. The socially disadvantaged position of Puerto Ricans is particularly apparent in their significant housing and health disparities.

The Housing Situation of Older Puerto Ricans

Older Puerto Ricans, like other older ethnic minority persons, experience significant housing inequality (Aguirre & Turner, 1995). Factors associated with oppression, including low socioeconomic status (SES), discrimination, and residential segregation, are primary contributors to their poor housing conditions. The 2000 U.S. Census depicts a precarious socioeconomic profile for many older Puerto Ricans, which can severely limit their ability to afford adequate housing. In 1999, 24.4% of Puerto Ricans 65 and over were below the poverty level with more women (26.6%) than men (19.6%) experiencing poverty.

Older Puerto Ricans receiving benefits from pensions and/or social security (benefits that often do not provide adequate income and reflect gender disparities), live well below the general standard of living for older persons. For example, 8.7% of all Puerto Ricans receive retirement incomes, with a mean value of $13,090; this compares to 16.7% of the general population with a mean value of $17,376. Many older Puerto Ricans worked as skilled blue collar and un-·skilled laborers holding jobs that had no retirement benefits. Some migrating late in life might not have accrued eligibility time or found jobs on the mainland. Clearly, poverty or scarce financial resources can be a major limiting factor in gaining equitable access to housing, particularly in an environment characterized by spiraling housing costs and tight market conditions with high demand for housing and low supply (Mutchler & Krivo, 1989).

Census data (2001) show that older Puerto Ricans are less likely to own a home (38.4%) than older persons in the larger population (78%), resulting in a disproportionate renter-to-owner ratio (61.6% renters: 38.4% owners vs. 22% renters: 78% owners). This exemplifies how homeownership, usually viewed as the cornerstone of the American dream, remains beyond their grasp (Mutchler & Krivo, 1989). Yet, homeownership is particularly important for older adults because of its inflation-protection benefits, and at this stage of the life cycle, assets and savings are expected to constitute a significant share of income portfolios (Flippen, 2001). Disparities also exist in terms of mortgage payments with more than 30% of older Puerto Ricans paying greater than 35% of their monthly income on such payment compared to only 16.3% of older adults in the general population.

Beyond severe affordability constraints, inequitable access to housing among older Puerto Ricans is likely to have been marked by residential segregation. In a study of national trends in Hispanic residential patterns, Logan (2002) found that Puerto Ricans were highly segregated from Whites and Blacks in a number of cities including New York City, which for many was historically the original entry point to the mainland. The index of disparity for Puerto Ricans was 56.5, which means that 56.5% of either Puerto Ricans or Whites would need to move to a new geographic area for the two groups to become equally distributed. For their aging members, living in segregated neighborhoods might have entailed limited opportunities across their lifespan in the labor market, education, and health care, setting the stage for their current disturbing sociodemographic profile. Confinement to specific geographic spaces can reduce access to spatially-determined resources, further blocking housing opportunities and restricting neighborhood options (Aguirre & Turner, 1995).

Residential segregation is closely interrelated to housing discrimination. Although it was outlawed in 1968, anti-discriminatory policies that regulate lending and real estate practices have not always been strongly enforced. Prejudicial policies of some financial and real estate institutions often pose barriers to procuring housing loans and direct customers to *appropriate* neighborhoods based on their ethnic and/or racial characteristics (Schaefer, 1996). Selling or renting solely based on personal prejudices and discrimination against members of certain ethnic groups still continues. In a qualitative study on culture and ethnicity in family caregiving (Ramos, 2001), Puerto Ricans related that landlords and real estate agents had limited their housing options to areas with large numbers of Hispanic residents while making it difficult to buy or rent in more desirable, primarily white, neighborhoods. Dark-skinned Puerto Ricans noted experiences of housing discrimination, which they attributed to prejudicial attitudes toward being Puerto Rican and Black. As low socioeconomic status (SES) and housing discrimination converge, many aging Puerto Ricans have found themselves without the security of homeownership, living in substandard housing conditions in segregated neighborhoods.

Over time, Puerto Ricans have formed separate distinct residential enclaves, or *barrios,* in disperse urban areas that have become identified as unique Puerto Rican communities (Canabal & Quiles, 1995). Logan (2002) reports their tendency to live in neighborhoods that are typically over 20% Puerto Rican. However, whether the tendency to settle in these enclaves is a determinant or a consequence of segregation is not clear, given that institutional racism, prejudice, and discrimination permeate throughout many aspects of their life experiences.

The *barrios* offer Puerto Rican older adults opportunities to reaffirm their ethnic identity and sense of pride, as well as a place from which to draw strength and resilience for survival in oppressive environments (Ramos, Toseland, McCallion, & Betancourt, 2004). Here, primarily through back and forth migration, some elements of Puerto Rican culture are maintained, readapted, and revitalized. As such, for many older adults, low SES, racism, and proximity to their only kin and other social networks, makes the *barrio* the only available option, although, at times, not necessarily the most desirable, preferred one.

Despite its multiple benefits, this residential pattern entails significant housing disadvantages. It often limits older Puerto Ricans to segregated, unsafe neighborhoods that need significant improvement in the cost and condition of housing. Moreover, their housing is likely to be smaller, of substandard quality, and more heavily rental (Krivo, 1995; Schaefer, 1996). Residential discrimination can be especially challenging for Puerto Ricans who are Black as they may be relegated close to African American neighborhoods where they may be isolated not only from the dominant group but also from the Puerto Rican, or broader Latino *barrios* (Aguirre & Turner, 1995).

The Health of Older Puerto Ricans

Research also provides a bleak picture of the overall health status for Puerto Rican older adults that is characterized by poor health status and caregiving needs marked by high rates of disability and dependency (Villa & Torres-Gil, 2001). As a result, older Puerto Ricans are likely to need significant care. For example, 65% of older Puerto Ricans in a national sample (Burnette & Mui, 1995) and 91.4% in a study in the northeast (Delgado & Tennstedt, 1997) reported their health to be poor to fair. In addition, older Puerto Ricans have a high prevalence of functional disability. The U.S. Census (2001) shows 55.1% of Puerto Ricans aged 65 or older have a disability compared to 44.1% of the general population. Delgado and Tennstedt (1997) found that 58% of the older adults in their study reported at least one functional disability. Using data from a national health study, Trevino and Moss (1984) found older Puerto Ricans (58%) were more likely to have more functional limitation in any activity than Whites (49%) and other older Latinos (Mexican Americans, 55% and Cubans, 47%). In this study, 50% of the Puerto Rican older women had limitation in major activity compared to White (34%), Mexican American (44%), and Cuban (37%) women.

The poor health status and high levels of functional disability found among older Puerto Ricans may be outcomes of their employment experiences, which are likely to have included physically taxing occupations and debilitating work conditions (Villa & Torres-Gil, 2001). Genetic, lifestyle, and environmental factors make them especially vulnerable to certain serious chronic conditions, such as diabetes, and its multiple medical and psychosocial complications (Aranda & Knight, 1997).

A Massachusetts study (Tucker, Bermudez, & Castaneda, 2000) found a higher diabetes rate for older Puerto Ricans (38.3% compared to 23.3% for White older adults) with a higher prevalence for women (40.4%) than men (35.5%). Further, as with other older Latinos, Puerto Ricans have earlier onset, more severe forms of the condition, and higher rates of complications, including kidney failure, blindness, and loss of limbs (Villa & Torres-Gil, 2001). These considerable health disparities are compounded by enduring disparities in health care, which have been attributed to multiple factors, including biases, stereotyping, and uncertainty on the part of the healthcare system (Talamantes & Aranda, 2004).

Despite their great health care needs, older Puerto Ricans typically benefit minimally from formal services (Mui & Burnette, 1994; Tennstedt, Chang, & Delgado, 1998). For example, families rarely use nursing homes or institutionalize an older relative and in 1999, only 3% of older Puerto Ricans were living in an institution (Mui & Burnette, 1994; U.S. Census, 2001). A study of older Puerto Ricans found that only 16.1% were recipients of formal long-term care services (Delgado & Tennstedt, 1997). Thus, serious questions are raised about the impact of health care disparities on the care of older Puerto Ricans, particularly as it appears to be taking place with little or no formal assistance whether in the context of institutional care, within an independent setting, or as a supplement to family caregiving.

LIVING ARRANGEMENTS AND CAREGIVING: THE ETHNOCULTURAL CONTEXTS

Puerto Ricans, like other Latinos, have historically shown a pattern of multigenerational co-residence most often attributed to cultural traditions and/or as a strategy to help offset the devastating consequences of poverty and limited housing options (Burr & Mutchler, 1999; Zsembik, 1996). The concept of familism can be useful in understanding this pattern as its practices facilitate the appropriate dynamics for extended family living arrangements and caregiving for older kin. Familism embodies the structural phenomenon of a shared household (Wallace & Facio, 1987) where aging members typically reside and receive care in the homes of adult children or other closely related kin. Its emphasis on reciprocity, cooperation, and interdependence fosters the development of strong family bonds and creates normative obligations among members, particularly older adults (Canino & Canino, 1993). Ideally, older adults are embedded within strong, hierarchical multigenerational family households where they are cared for and enjoy a high status due to ascription and recognition of their valuable life-long experience (Ramos et al., 2004).

Traditional familism emerged at a different time and place, and its practices, which help make co-residence feasible, are becoming increasingly more challenging in today's society (Purdy & Arguello, 1992). As Puerto Rican families continue to adapt to mainland sociocultural conditions, structural forces, particularly in light of significant housing and economic disadvantages, may override their ability to preserve familism practices that ease co-residence and the care for aging relatives (Tennstedt et al., 1998). Culture change, opportunities, and resources differentially influence Puerto Ricans' living arrangements.

Like their aging members, Puerto Rican families tend to live in small, substandard, crowded residences in poor inner-city neighborhoods (Aguirre & Turner, 1995), and have an overall household poverty level of 23.4% and 28% for households with children under 18 (U.S. Census, 2001) that severely limits their ability to afford better housing. Despite efforts, many families may not be able to provide adequate living conditions for co-residing older members, particularly since they are likely to be highly disabled and require home modifications. Some older adults may need to use ramps, rails, and ground floor accommodations that may be nearly impossible to afford or implement given limited living space that must be shared among all family members. Thus, providing care with minimal formal supports can compromise its effectiveness in meeting the older person's proper living conditions and physical and emotional well-being (Purdy & Arguello, 1992). To secure an appropriate living environment and caregiving conditions for older Puerto Ricans within a co-residence setting, many families still need formal assistance and adequate, ·affordable housing.

Although for some older Puerto Ricans, co-residency and its associated family caregiving are a reality; for others, this type of living arrangement may not always be an option. The structure and gender roles of Puerto Rican families are changing as a result of socioeconomic adaptation to the mainland (Delgado & Tennstedt, 1997). As such, the presence of large, multigenerational households to provide co-residency and care for aging kin may not be as pervasive today. According to the U.S. Census (2001) Puerto Ricans have a mean household size of 2.97 compared to 3.90 for Mexican Americans and 2.48 for non-Latino whites. Also, 17.4% of Puerto Rican households have five or more persons compared to 34.7% for Mexican Americans and 8.8% for non-Latino whites, and a high rate of single-parent households (46%). Interestingly, among older Puerto Rican women co-residing with others, 31.5% maintain headship compared to 16.2% of their White counterparts (Burr & Mutchler, 1999).

Acculturation, economic factors, and recent social trends have contributed to this tendency toward smaller households and other changes that reduce their availability for coresidency and caregiving (Tennstedt et al., 1998). For example, more acculturated offspring may have adopted mainstream values that do not emphasize co-residency and filial piety as strongly (Delgado & Tennstedt, 1997). Also, employment opportunities may require large geographic distance between adult children and parents, reducing the potential for multigenerational households for caregiving. Again, families willing to share their homes with aging kin may be impeded by the realities of their own substandard housing and economic situations. For some older persons, back-and-forth migration may have disrupted the continuity of family relationships, reducing the number of potential family households available for co-residency (Delgado & Tennstedt, 1997).

A likely shortage of available families for co-residency may partially explain the current pattern of living arrangements of older Puerto Ricans. Only a relatively low percentage (30%) was living with an extended family member other than a spouse (U.S. Census, 2001). De Vos and Arias (2003) documented a decrease in the rate of older Puerto Ricans co-residing with an adult child from 40% in 1980 to 28% in 2000. Moreover, contrary to popular notions about the pervasiveness of older minority persons living in multigenerational households, older Puerto Ricans are more likely to live alone (30%) or with only a spouse (34%). Here, gender ratio differences are clear, as it is mostly older women (67.5%) who are more likely to be living alone (U.S. Census, 2001). Older

Puerto Ricans also show a steady trend toward living independently, from 25% living alone in 1970 to the current 30% (De Vos & Arias, 2003). This trend reflects some pronounced changes when compared to other Latinos, particularly Mexican Americans, who remained at 20% living alone from 1970 to 2000. For Puerto Ricans, the number of couple-only households has also grown from 19% in 1970 to today's 34%.

These changes in living arrangements may also be due to personal preferences. For example, data from the National Survey of Hispanic Elderly People (Zsembik, 1996) indicate that 86.8% of Puerto Rican older adults who live alone reported preferring it to co-residency. The more acculturated might have adopted mainland values such as individualism, self-reliance, and independence that underlie the preference for living alone or in a nuclear household (Ramos, 1997).

For others, living independently may not necessarily reflect a dramatic change in value systems, a desirable choice, or the result of a free-will decision but a necessary response to environmental pressures. For instance, some of these older persons may deliberately cede opportunities to co-reside with their children because of sadness and concerns about becoming a burden and fear of interfering with their progress (Zsembick, 1996; Ramos, 2004). Zsembick (1996) suggests that Puerto Ricans may become accustomed at an early age to the lifestyle associated with living in single adult households because of the prevalence of female-headed households in this population. Hence, there appears to be a discrepancy between strong attitudes favoring this type of living arrangement and actual behaviors, as evidenced by the relatively low rate of co-residency among older Puerto Ricans and their families. Hence, familism norms that specifically prescribe co-residence are being challenged, calling attention to accompanying changes in caregiving patterns.

Puerto Rican families who do not co-reside with their aging members have not automatically rescinded their filial responsibility, which is strongly emphasized by familism norms of reciprocity to provide care. Data on attitudes about intergenerational filial responsibility show a stronger commitment among Latinos than non-Latino Whites (Burr & Mutchler, 1999; Goldschneider & Lawton, 1998). In fact, Puerto Rican families continue to play an essential role in the caregiving of their aging members (Delgado & Tennstedt, 1997). It should be noted, however, that Puerto Rican families appear to be adopting new, less traditional, caregiving strategies that suggest a continued willingness to provide care for aging kin even when unable or available to do so through co-residency. A study in Springfield, Massachusetts, found that Puerto Rican kin, predominantly women, who were not residing with their aging relative, were providing caregiving even though it involved much traveling and, in a sense, maintaining two households (Tennstedt et al., 1998). Here, 77% reported seeing them at least daily (Delgado & Tennstedt, 1997).

At the same time, questions have been raised over the quality and quantity of care these families can provide within this type of living arrangement, given competing responsibilities and often adverse housing and socioeconomic conditions. Research indicates that offspring who do not co-reside with their older kin provide less care than other caregivers, and in particular, with help that is more intensive, tangible, hands-on assistance such as day-to-day necessary care (Delgado & Tennstedt, 1997). Further, limited housing options often preclude close proximity or increased opportunities for older persons to enjoy a much predicated, perhaps, long-anticipated, special status ascribed by the value of familism. Thus, despite a willingness and effort to practice familism norms of filial piety, doing so in separate residential settings may not have optimal consequences for older Puerto Ricans.

Concerns have also been raised about the impact of living independently on older Puerto Ricans for whom family supports are virtually non-existent. In general, older adults who live alone are less likely to have reliable informal support systems, and Puerto Ricans, particularly women, may be especially vulnerable due to their housing, health, and economic disadvantages (Burnette & Mui, 1995). Their already worrisome predicament is often exacerbated by the tendency to make little use of some long-term care formal services such as home health aides and meals on wheels programs (Burnette & Mui, 1995; Wallace & Villa, 1999). In sum, the changing patterns of living arrangements and caregiving among older Puerto Ricans have important implications for housing policy.

AGING IN PLACE AND OLDER PUERTO RICANS

On the U.S. mainland, prevailing attitudes about the appropriateness of housing older adults in special shelter and residential care facilities are shifting toward a greater recognition of the living environment preference of older people to stay where they are and *age in place* (Houben, 2001; Prosper, Sherman, & Howe, 2000). From this perspective, older persons are enabled to remain in their own familiar surroundings longer by providing them with care in a housing setting.

Houben (2001) identifies two approaches to aging in place. The first approach involves structural adaptation of the home and living environment, often making use of home technology, which allows people to function independently longer. Basic facilities are available within a very short distance. Optimally, an older person does not have to move, or not until the last stages of life, as the care that is taking place at home can be increased as needed.

The second approach comes into play when the first approach cannot be implemented properly or when an older person cannot continue living at home and moving to a residential facility is the only option. In this facility a flexible combination of resources to support self-reliance are made available as needed so that future moves will not be required. For a given older person, the most suitable approach to aging in place is contingent upon individual housing situations, economic conditions, and health care needs.

Aging in place is a western concept based on the values of autonomy, privacy, and the right to make individual choices. Efforts to implement the concept are relatively recent (Houben, 2001), although the notion of a person growing old within familiar surroundings rather than in an institution has been in existence cross-culturally for a considerable time. For Puerto Ricans, it is consistent with familism norms that ascribe members a stable place in the family where they can be cared for as they grow old. Further, placing an older member in an institution is not culturally sanctioned and virtually prohibited.

At the same time, this western conceptualization of aging in place, and the ways in which it is implemented, could be expanded to accommodate changing patterns of living arrangements and closely related approaches to care for older Puerto Ricans. For example, older adults co-residing with extended families could readily use some of the formal supports and home modification strategies. Those who live independently could still benefit from the involvement of kin committed to familism norms of filial piety to complement formal services. Similarly, drawing upon other informal support systems to offset and gradually incorporate reliance on formal services should be considered.

Society's attitudinal changes, economic factors, and cultural preferences have sparked interest among policymakers and program developers for whom assisting older persons to age in place is a way to improve the older adult's quality of life as well as save federal and state government resources (Heuman, Winter-Nelson, & Anderson, 2001).

For example, Section 202 Supportive Housing for the Elderly Program, Section 8 housing, Hope for Elderly Independence, and the Congregate Housing Services Program serve as a bulwark of independence for older persons. These programs, directly or indirectly, support at least some aspects of aging in place. Yet, given disadvantaged housing conditions, changing patterns of living arrangements and related approaches to care, how appropriate these policies are in assisting older Puerto Ricans to successfully realize their vision of aging in place is unclear. A discussion of the relevance of Section 202 and recommendations that could help increase its appropriateness as a viable program in assisting older Puerto Ricans to move closer to their vision of aging in place follows.

THE SECTION 202 SUPPORTIVE HOUSING
FOR THE ELDERLY PROGRAM

Section 202 was originally authorized in the National Housing Act of 1959 and its financing and mission have been modified several times. To be eligible, a person must be at least 62 years of age with an income that is 50% below that of the median income in the local area. In 1999, 5,000 housing projects with over 260,000 units were created, and more than 300,000 older persons were housed in over 3,500 Section 202 facilities (Heuman et al., 2001). Section 202 is considered the single most successful Federal housing program for older persons. Because it provides affordable residential accommodations as well as supportive services, it can be a potential vehicle for older persons with low incomes to age in place.

The increasing trend toward living independently, high poverty rates, and limited housing alternatives make the Section 202 program, at least in principle, especially relevant for Puerto Rican older adults, given their distinct ethnocultural realities. Although this program does not address the predicament of co-residing older persons, with some provisions it can strengthen its cultural congruency for older Puerto Ricans who are increasingly living independently.

First, data from the 1999 American Association of Retired Person's (AARP) study of the Section 202 program, which depicts the status of the program's residential facilities (Heuman et al., 2001) helps identify some areas that could be addressed to increase suitability for older Puerto Ricans. For example, units are typically constructed as private studios or one-bedroom apartments. More two bedrooms apartments are needed as these could accommodate a family caregiver or another member of the older person's informal support system on a permanent or temporary basis. Yet, only 1.2% of existing apartments have two bedrooms with 83.1% one bedroom and 15.5% efficiencies (Heuman et al., 2001).

Also, residents in general could benefit from additional space in the communal area. This could facilitate interaction with visiting family members, which for some older Puerto Ricans may occur often and include large numbers of visitors at once. Further, intergenerational centers would enhance the quality of their day-to-day experiences. Similarly, among older Puerto Ricans, playing dominos and other table games in groups is a very common leisure time activity. Currently, most facilities (90.2%) have one multi-purpose, social/recreational activity space, and some (50%) also have a congregate dining room (Heuman et al., 2001). This arrangement may be considered appropriate to meet the needs of mainstream older persons who may be more likely to prefer the privacy of their own apartments, but changes are needed to meet the living environment preferences of ethnically diverse residents.

Some building complexes in the metropolitan areas and larger cities are located in neighborhoods with high crime rates where violence, gangs, and drugs are common. Here, effective strategies are needed to create partnerships with community representatives, including gang leaders, to secure the residents' safety. An AARP study found that buildings located in the larger cities and metropolitan areas had the greatest proportion of minority residents, suggesting their greater risk for unsafe living situations (Heuman et al., 2001). For older Puerto Ricans this predicament is especially relevant given that, in 1999, 97% lived in urban settings (U.S. Census, 2001).

Additionally, support services must be culturally appropriate. For example, congregate meals should include dishes that are consistent with Puerto Rican diet and cuisine. Special attention should be given to language preferences; culturally bound concepts of illness, wellness, and syndromes; and natural healing systems. Further, service providers might include faith-based organizations such as the Pentecostal Church, which also offers instrumental assistance to its members and is becoming increasingly popular among Puerto Ricans, particularly older adults (Delgado, 1996). The above recommendations are not meant to be exhaustive but to provide a starting point.

Despite its potential to address pressing housing and caregiving needs within the context of aging in place, the impact of Section 202 on the lives of older Puerto Ricans has been minimal. For example, although specific figures for older Puerto Ricans are not available, Hispanic residents of Section 202 facilities comprised only 5%, compared to 4.5% for Asians, 75.9% non-Latino Whites, and 13.6% African Americans. In fact, from 1988 to 1999 Latinos remained at 5% while African Americans and Asians increased from 11.5% to 13.6% and 1.5% to 4.5%, respectively (Heuman et al., 2001). This is surprising since Latinos have been steadily growing in numbers, and today are the largest ethnic minority group. It is possible that information about the program is not reaching this population due to language and geographic barriers, factors identified in the under-utilization of formal services (Dietz, 1997).

Prejudicial attitudes and discriminatory behaviors may have also contributed to their potential under-representation among Section 202 program participants. Some older Puerto Ricans, and their families, might not have considered this type of housing because they felt discouraged at the prospect of not being able to share living space with at least one extended family member. Perhaps they feared feeling like outsiders when they were the only Latino residents in the facility and in an almost foreign environment. Clearly, all of these potential impediments can and should be successfully addressed. In general, less funding and a high demand for Section 202 units, with long waiting lists, limits the ability of this program to meet the needs of many older adults with low incomes. Nonetheless, the potential under-representation of Puerto Ricans and other Latinos is still disconcerting.

CONCLUSION

As the U.S. older population becomes increasingly diversified, it is incumbent on the social work profession to advocate for policies and programs that address the housing needs of older persons in traditionally neglected, highly vulnerable oppressed populations, including Puerto Ricans. Yet, as Wallace and Villa (1999) point out, the needs of minority older adults remain *invisible* in the public arena where they are buffeted by policy changes that do not take them into account. This invisibility, particularly in the areas of housing and health, is due, in part, to generalizations that depict all minority older persons as living in multigenerational family households where they receive care and, therefore, formal supports are not needed (Bengston, Rosenthal, & Burton, 1995).

Understanding the ethno-cultural realities of both older adults who co-reside in multigenerational households and those who live independently is essential to policy formation and program planning. Formal services to address their housing and caregiving needs, whether as a supplement to family caregiving, within an independent context, or in the form of institutional care, are an entitlement that is long overdue. Housing policy should facilitate and support the traditional family caregiving tendencies among Puerto Ricans or any cultural group and avoid creating incentives that could thwart or undermine such tendencies.

A prudent policy direction should be in the expansion of programs supporting at-home care. Currently states and localities have incentives to use Medicaid money for institutional care. A wiser policy direction would include expanded opportunities to use public health dollars for at-home care. With the obvious benefits associated with shared living, there might be a role for expanded definitions of families or households when determining benefit eligibility. Family and community members should be eligible to receive financial support for caregiving as a way to avoid institutionalization.

Concerns regarding future availability of family co-residency and the trend toward independent residency among some groups such as Puerto Ricans call for more culturally relevant social and economic policies to maintain this type of living arrangement. Policymakers should continue to support the provision of housing subsidies for the elderly. As noted with regard to Section 202, constructing larger units to accommodate kin caregivers and provide more communal space could better meet the housing needs of ethnically diverse elders. Given the dependence of many generations on public housing (Zsembick, 1996), policy makers could make provisions for residents to move into larger units to facilitate older kin opportunities for co-residence. For older adults, current regulations restricting the number of residents per unit limit their opportunities to co-reside.

Future policies addressing community planning could include the construction of larger housing units. Perhaps there could be policy incentives in that direction for communities and individuals (such as tax incentives for "mother-in-law" or, perhaps, "family-in-law" apartments being included in new housing construction). Communities could be planned around pedestrian-friendly easy travel and short trips, rather than as suburban sprawl. Financing could be made available to build and rehabilitate housing to help preserve and revitalize the *barrios* and end displacement. An adequate housing policy must end racial/ethnic discrimination that leads to housing segregation through affirmative housing programs and a more vigorous enforcement of fair housing laws (Karger & Stoesz, 2002). Ideally, the opportunity to live in adequate housing in familiar healthy, and safe neighborhoods should become a right rather than a privilege available equally to older adults of all racial and ethnic backgrounds.

An important consideration is the development of housing policies that provide underserved older adults with a full range of services options, including community-based programs, which are congruent with their own vision of aging in place. As such, these must take into account their historical disadvantaged housing conditions, current and changing patterns of living arrangements, and related caregiving practices. Policies should include provisions mandating that programs address structural and cultural barriers previously reported in the literature (Wallace & Villa, 1999).

Providing culturally competent housing services is consistent with the social work profession's charge (NASW, 2001). As such, it is critical to develop appropriate outreach strategies, and services must be accessible, affordable, and linguistically and culturally relevant. For example, social service agencies could be encouraged to develop stronger ties with existing community-based services and more actively recruit historically underserved older adults. Information about existing formal services for older adults, health, transportation, and financial assistance in their home language should be made readily available. It is essential to expand the staff's racial/ethnic diversity, and hold regular mandated sensitivity trainings that highlight the need to recognize cross-cultural differences in family structures and preferred living arrangements.

Of utmost importance, assumptions about a preference and availability of kin for co-residence among older adults of certain racial/ethnic groups, namely Puerto Ricans, must be reevaluated as this can directly impinge upon the effectiveness of housing services. The 21st century, with its rising aging populations offers new opportunities to redress institutional ethnic and racial barriers to housing rights for older Puerto Ricans. Disparities in access to aging in place services and supports must be rectified.

REFERENCES

Aguirre, A., & Turner, J. (1995). *American ethnicity: The dynamics and consequences of discrimination*. New York: McGraw Hill.

Aranda, M., & Knight, B. (1997). The influence of ethnicity and culture on caregivers. *The Gerontologist, 37*(3), 342-357.

Bengtson, V., Rosenthal, C., & Burton, L. (1995). Paradoxes of families and aging. In: R. Binstock & L. George (Eds), *Handbook of Aging and the Social Sciences*, pp. 254-282. San Diego: Academic Press.

Burnette, D., & Mui, A. (1995). In-home and community-based service utilization by three groups of elderly Hispanics. *Social Work Research, 19*(4), 197-206.

Burr, J., & Mutchler, J. (1992). The living arrangements of unmarried elderly Hispanic females. *Demography, 29*, 93-112.

Burr, J., & Mutchler, J. (1999). Race and ethnic variation in norms of filial responsibility among older persons. *Journal of Marriage and the Family, 61*(3), 674-687.

Canabal, M., & Quiles, J. (1995). Acculturation and socioeconomic factors as determinants of depression among Puerto Ricans in the United States. *Social Behavior and Personality, 23*(3), 235-248.

Canino, I., & Canino, G. (1993). Psychiatric care of Puerto Ricans. In. A. Gaw (Ed.), *Culture, Ethnicity, and Mental Illness*. Washington, D.C.: American Psychiatric Press.

Delgado, M., & Tennstedt, S. (1997). Making the case for culturally appropriate community services: Puerto Rican elders and their caregivers. *Health and Social Work, 22*, 246-255.

Delgado, M. (1996). Religion as a caregiving system for Puerto Rican elders with functional disabilities. *Journal of Gerontological Social Work, 26*, 129-144.

DeVos, S., & Arias, E. (2003). A note on living arrangements of elders 1970-1999, with special emphasis on Hispanic subgroup differentials. *Population Research and Policy Review, 22*, 91-101.

Dietz, C. (2000). Responding to oppression and violence: A feminist challenge to clinical social work. *Affilia, 15*(3), 369-389.

Flippen, C. (2001). Racial and ethnic inequality in homeownership and housing equity. *The Sociological Quarterly, 42*(2), 121-149.

Goldschneider, F., & Lawton, L. (1998). Family experiences and the erosion of support for intergenerational coresidence. *Marriage and the Family, 60*, 623-632.

Heumann, L., Winter-Nelson, K., & Anderson, J. (2001). *The 1999 national survey of Section 202 Elderly Housing–Executive Summary*. American Association of Retired Persons (AARP). *htpp://research.aarp.org*.

Houben, P. (2001). Changing housing for elderly people and co-ordination issues in Europe. *Housing Studies, 16*(5), 651-673.

Karger, H., & Stoesz, D. (2002). American social welfare policy: A pluralist approach. Boston, MA: Allyn and Bacon.

Krivo, L. (1995). Immigrant characteristics and Hispanic-Anglo housing inequality. *Demography, 32*(4), 599-615.

Logan, J. (2002). Hispanic Populations and Their Residential Patterns in the Metropolis. *Lewis Mumford Center for Comparative Urban and Regional Research*. University at Albany, State University of New York.

Mui, A., & Burnette, D. (1994). Long-term care service use by frail elders: Is ethnicity a factor? *The Gerontologist, 34*(2), 190-198.

Mutchler, J., & Krivo, L. (1989). Availability and affordability: Household adaptation to a housing squeeze. *Social Forces, 68*(1), 241-261.

National Association of Social Workers. (2001). *Standards for Cultural Competence in Social Work Practice*. Silver Springs, MD. NASW Press.

Parrillo, V. (2002). *Strangers to these shores*. Boston: Allyn and Bacon.

Pearlin, L., Mullan, J., Semple, S., & Skall, M (1990). Caregiving and the stress process: An overview of concepts and their measures. *The Gerontologist, 30*, 583-594.

Prosper, V., Sherman, S., & Howe, J. (2000). Living arrangements for older New Yorkers. In *Project 2015: The future of aging in New York State* (pp. 35-41). Albany: The New York State Office for the Aging.

Purdy, J., & Arguello, D. (1992). Hispanic familism in caretaking of older adults: Is it functional? *Journal of Gerontological Social Work, 19*, 29-43.

Ramos, B. (1997). Acculturation and depression among Puerto Ricans and Puerto Rican veterans in the Continental U.S. *Doctoral Dissertation*, U of Albany, New York.

Ramos, B. (2001). Parenting, caregiver stress, and child abuse and neglect. In A. Sallee, H. Lawson, and K. Briar-Lawson (Eds.), *Innovative practices with vulnerable children and families* (pp. 209-228). Dubuque, IA: Eddie Bowers Publishing.

Ramos, B. Toseland, R., McCallion, P., & Betancourt, D. (2004). Caregiving in Latino Families: The Roles of Cultural and Social Factors. Paper presented at the 54th Annual Scientific Meeting of the Gerontological Society of America. Chicago, IL. November 2001.

Ramos, B. (2004). Culture, ethnicity, and caregiver stress among Puerto Ricans. *Journal of Applied Gerontology. 23*(4), 469-486.

Ramos, B., Jones, L., & Toseland, R. (2005). Social work practice with older adults of color. In: D. Lum (Ed.), *Cultural Competence, Practice Stages, and Client Systems* (pp. 320-358). Australia: Brooks Cole.

Rivera-Batiz, R., & Santiago, C. (1994). *Puerto Ricans in the United States: A changing reality*. Washington, D.C.: The National Puerto Rican Coalition.

Schaefer, R. (1996). *Racial and Ethnic Groups*. New York: HarperCollins.

Talamantes, M., & Aranda, M. (2004). *Cultural competency in working with Latino family caregivers*. San Francisco: Family Caregiver Alliance.

Tennstedt, S., Chang, B., & Delgado, M. (1998). Patterns of long-term care: Comparison of Puerto Rican, African-American, and Non-Latino White caregivers. In M. Delgado (Ed.), *Latino elders and the twenty-first century: Issues and challenges for culturally competent research and practice* (pp. 179-200). NY: Haworth.

Trevino, F., & Moss, A. (1984). Health indicators for Hispanic, Black, and White Americans. *Vital Statistics, 10*, 148-188.

Tucker, K., Bermudez, O., & Castaneda, C. (2000). Type 2 diabetes is prevalent and poorly controlled among Hispanics of Caribbean origin. *Family Relations, 90*(8), 1288-1293.

United States Bureau of the Census. (2001). *Hispanic population in the United States. Current Population Survey*. Washington, D.C.: U.S. Government Printing Office.

Villa, V., & Torres-Gil, F. (2001). The later years: The health of elderly Latinos. In: M. Aguirre-Molina, C. Mollilna, & R. Zambrana (Eds.), *Health Issues in the Latino Community* (pp. 157-178). San Francisco: Jossey-Bass.

Wallace, S., & Facio, E. (1987). Moving beyond familism: Potential contributions of gerontological theory to studies of chicano/latino aging. *Journal of Aging Studies, 1*, 337-354.

Wallace, S., & Villa, V. (1999). Caught in hostile cross-fire: Public policy and minority elderly in the United States. In K. Markides & M. Miranda (Eds.), *Aging, Health, and Ethnicity* (pp. 237-255). Thousand Oaks: Sage.

Wilmoth, J. (2001). Living arrangements among older immigrants in the United States. *The Gerontologist, 42*(2), 228-328.

Zsembick, B. (1996). Preference for coresidence among older Latinos. *Journal of Aging Studies, 10*(1), 69-81.

doi:10.1300/J083v49n01_03

Challenges
for Grandparent Housing Programs

Stacey R. Kolomer, PhD
Karen Y. Lynch, LMSW

SUMMARY. The purpose of this article is to explore the current and developing grandparent caregiver housing programs throughout the United States. Telephone interviews were conducted with eight current and proposed sites for grandparent and/or relative caregivers throughout the United States. Housing design, funding sources, referral sources, service provided, and rules and regulations of the housing programs were discussed. Funding, education, and advocacy appeared crucial to helping these families provide safe homes for the children in their care. Recommendations are made for social workers and grandparent caregivers to lobby legislators for increases in funding for programs nationwide to ensure all grandparent families have safe, affordable and accessible housing. doi:10.1300/J083v49n01_04 *[Article copies available for a fee from The Haworth Document Delivery Service: 1-800-HAWORTH. E-mail address: <docdelivery@haworthpress.com> Website: <http://www.HaworthPress.com> © 2007 by The Haworth Press, Inc. All rights reserved.]*

KEYWORDS. Grandparent caregivers, housing

[Haworth co-indexing entry note]: "Challenges for Grandparent Housing Programs." Kolomer, Stacey R., and Karen Y. Lynch. Co-published simultaneously in *Journal of Gerontological Social Work* (The Haworth Press, Inc.) Vol. 49, No. 1/2, 2007, pp. 65-79; and: *Housing for the Elderly: Policy and Practice Issues* (ed: Philip McCallion) The Haworth Press, Inc., 2007, pp. 65-79. Single or multiple copies of this article are available for a fee from The Haworth Document Delivery Service [1-800-HAWORTH, 9:00 a.m. - 5:00 p.m. (EST). E-mail address: docdelivery@haworthpress.com].

Available online at http://jgsw.haworthpress.com
© 2007 by The Haworth Press, Inc. All rights reserved.
doi:10.1300/J083v49n01_04

INTRODUCTION

Grandparents' homes have been called "the second line of defense" or the "safety net" for children when a temporary crisis occurs in a family (Kornhaber, 1986; Minkler, Roe, & Price, 1992). However, for increasing numbers of children, grandparents and other relatives have become their permanent caregivers. Approximately 6.3% of all children in the United States are living in grandparent-headed households, and in one-third of these homes the children's parents are not present (Emick & Hayslip, 1999; Fuller-Thomson & Minkler, 2000; Fuller-Thomson, Minkler, & Driver, 1997; Silverstein & Vehvilainen, 1998). The U.S. Census Bureau (2002) reports that from 1990 to 1997 kinship caregiver households increased by 31% and grandparent-only households increased by 27%. Presently one in ten grandparents will take on the role of primary caregiver to a grandchild for at least six months before the child is 18 years old (Burnette, 1999; Silverstein & Vehvilainen, 1998).

Becoming a permanent caregiver to one's grandchildren can have unexpected benefits as well as unwelcomed challenges. Caregiving for one's grandchildren can provide a purpose for living, and increase love and companionship, hope for the future, feelings of being appreciated, and satisfaction of helping others (Burton & deVries, 1992; Emick & Hayslip, 1996, 1999; Hayslip, Shore, Henderson, & Lambert, 1998; Jendrek, 1994; Kolomer & McCallion, 2005; Minkler & Roe, 1993; Minkler, Roe, & Price, 1992). Despite the many rewards that come from caregiving, grandparent caregivers also face many challenges. Some of the issues that grandparent caregivers must cope with include physical and mental health problems, emotional burnout, financial strain, and difficulty in finding safe, adequate, and affordable housing (Kolomer, McCallion, & Janicki, 2002).

The purpose of this article is to explore current and developing grandparent caregiver housing programs throughout the United States. This article will discuss the housing challenges for grandparent caregivers, offer a description of current and potential federal funding resources for the development of grandparent housing, and outline challenges for the current and developing model housing programs for grandparent caregivers nationwide. Overall, adequate, safe, affordable, and supportive housing for grandparent caregivers is imperative to improving the lives of these exceptional families (Kanders, 2002; Generations United, 2003).

HOUSING ISSUES FOR GRANDPARENT CAREGIVERS

U.S. Census (2000) has reported that 2.4 million grandparents are the primary caregivers for their grandchildren, and 39% of these grandparents have provided over 5 years of care to children under the age of 18 (Generations United, 2003). Becoming a grandparent caregiver has been associated with financial strain. According to a study conducted by the U.S. Census Bureau in 1997, approximately one in four (27%) grandparent-maintained households were impoverished (Casper & Bryson, 1998). Current empirical research on the Census 2000 Supplementary Survey discovered, "237,516 grandparent caregivers lived below the poverty line, which was $17,603/year for a family of four" (Fuller-Thompson & Minkler, 2003, p. 93; Dalaker, 2001). Further, 60% of grandparent caregivers are living below the poverty line and are not receiving any federal housing subsidies (Fuller-Thompson & Minkler, 2003).

In addition to the financial challenges, living space can also create problems for caregivers. Grandparents and other relatives often begin caring for children with little or no warning or preparation. Housing difficulties for grandparent caregivers include the following:

- The residence may be too small to accommodate more people;
- There may be overcrowding;
- Neighborhood may be unsafe and the caregiver may be unable to relocate due to finances;
- The presence of children may violate lease agreements;
- The residence may have safety hazards; and
- Housing is inadequately equipped for persons with physical challenges.

There has been very limited research about the housing conditions of grandparent caregivers. Fuller-Thomson and Minkler (2003) found that of the 2,350,000 grandparent caregivers in the United States in the year 2000

- a little over a quarter were renters and one third of these renters were spending more than 30% of their income on housing.
- 14% of the grandparent families lived in public housing.
- 3 out of 10 of the grandparent-headed households were living in overcrowded conditions.

Given the increase in grandparent-headed housholds, in 1988 the federal Fair Housing Act was amended to prohibit housing discrimination due to the presence of children. The only exception was for housing that was clearly defined as senior citizen (United States Department of Justice, 1994). Grandparents who reside in the senior citizen section of public housing or in senior apartments and become cargivers to their grandchildren may still therefore face eviction.

FEDERAL OPTIONS TO FUND HOUSING ALTERNATIVES

Despite the difficulties experienced with grandparent-headed households in regards to housing, there has been limited national policy developed to address this area of need. At the federal level there are several housing programs that have been used to fund alternative housing: Section 8 Vouchers, Hope VI, and CHDO. There has also been a proposed program, LEGACY, to expand funding options.

Section 8 Vouchers. Section 8 is a federal voucher and certificate program funded by the U.S. Department of Housing and Urban Development (HUD) (Bloom & Bloom, 1984). It is available to low income families, older adults, and people with disabilities (Technical Assistance Program, 2005). A Section 8 voucher enables members of a low income household to pay 30% of their income towards the rent of an apartment or house with HUD then paying the difference. The apartment must be a qualified home and rent for an amount that does not exceed HUD's Fair Market price for the area. If the home does rent for more than fair market for the area, the renter must pay the excess. Section 8 vouchers offer low-income renters greater choices of where to live. However, the waiting of list to qualify for Section 8 is sometimes as long as 4 years (Rental Housing Online, 2005). In addition, to qualify, the income of the household must typically be 50% or less of the area median income, with 75 percent of the vouchers being given to households with incomes below 30 percent of the area median income (Technical Assistance Program, 2005). The development of several grandparent housing options, e.g., Boston Grandfamilies House, has been possible through the specific allocation and pooling of Section 8 Vouchers.

Hope VI. The National Commission on Severely Distressed Public Housing developed a National Action Plan to eradicate severely distressed public housing (US Department of Housing and Urban Development, 2005). Launched in 1992, Hope VI's purpose was to eliminate severely distressed public housing by offering funding to Public Housing Authorities (HUD, 2005; Popkin, Katz, Cunningham, Brown, Gustafson, & Turner, 2004). Any public housing authority that has severely distressed housing units can apply for HOPE VI funding to revitalize those units. Money received from Hope VI can fund major rehabilitation, new construction, demolition of housing in severe distress, relocation, planning and technical assistance, management improvements, and community and supportive services for residents (US Department of Housing and Urban Development, 2005). Two Public Housing Authorities have utilized Hope VI to develop housing for grandparent caregiving families, Boston Housing Authority and Buffalo Housing Authority.

Community Housing Development Organization (CHDO). A CHDO is a private nonprofit organization with 501 (c) 3 federal tax exemptions whose purpose is to provide affordable housing for low income households. With the distinction of being a CHDO, organizations can then qualify for HOME funds. The purpose of HOME is to expand the supply of affordable housing, particularly for low-income citizens, to reinforce state and local governments' abilities to design and implement strategies and to support partnerships and collaboration between government, profit, and non-profit organizations to develop affordable housing (US Department of Housing and Urban Development, 2005). HOME supports local communities to develop types of housing which best suit their region, empowering the communities to create housing for its constituents. Six grandparent housing programs currently have or are waiting for CHDO status.

LEGACY. The LEGACY (Living Equitably: Grandparents Aiding Children and Youth) bill was signed into law December 16, 2003. This bill proposed to provide funding and opportunities for the replication of Grandfamilies House, a model grandparent housing unit. The intent of this bill is to allow grandparent families to qualify for the Section 8 Family Unification Program. In addition this bill would support grant funding for a national study of the housing needs of grandparents raising grandchildren, funding for the expansion of grandparent family homes, and educational training for Housing & Urban Development (HUD) workers about the uniqueness of grandparent families (Generations United, 2003). To date this Act has not received funding.

STUDY DESIGN

Sample: Telephone interviews were conducted with key staff at eight current and proposed sites for grandparent and/or relative caregivers throughout the United States. The sites were identified from web searches and contacts with national grandparent advocacy programs. Informants included the executive directors at each site, and the social services coordinator, project developer, director of community relations, and director of the grandparent units at specific sites.

Table 1 lists the eight sites and their stages of development. In 1998, Grandfamilies House in Boston, Massachusetts was the first housing program to respond to the challenges faced by grandparent-headed households. This intergenerational program provides housing and support services for children and grandparents. This program has been nationally recognized and other programs throughout the United States have been attempting to replicate its model.

Boston Grandfamilies House and Presbyterian Social Services Grandparent family apartments (PSS) serve only grandparent-headed households. Boston

TABLE 1. Grandparent Housing Units

Facility Name /Developer	City/State	Structure	Stage of Development
Grandfamilies/ Currently merging with Community Development Corporation due to financial concerns	Boston, Massachusetts	26 units two and three bedroom units with 2 baths and one 4 bedroom unit 3 bathrooms Apartments are in high rise buildings, with elevators and are wheelchair accessible.	Current Residents
Boston Housing Authority	Boston, Massachusetts	15 units 4 flats and 11 townhouses (2 and 3 bedrooms) all apartment are handicap accessible and can be modified as needed.	Current Residents
Buffalo Housing Authority	Buffalo, New York	17 townhomes all are handicap adaptable by lowering cabinets, modifying bathrooms	Current Residents
Casa Familia/ Casa Otonal	New Haven, Connecticut	1. Current facility is a three family house with grandparents raising grandchildren 2-3 bedrooms. 2. Families Currently building a new facility with 30 units of 16 two bedroom and 14 three bedrooms and to be modeled after Grandfamilies.	1. Current Residents 2. Construction Plan to open 2005
Grandparent Family Apartments/ Presbyterian Social Services	Bronx, New York	40 two bedroom and 10 three bedroom apartments with one two bedroom superintendent in a six story building with elevators.	Construction Plan to open at the end of 2004
Kinship Village/ Fairhill Center for Aging	Cleveland, Ohio	12 apartments specifically for grandparents caring for toddlers and young children.	Pre-construction Plan to open at the end of 2005
Elizabeth's Place/ Grandfamilies Housing Task Force	El Rino, Oklahoma	90-95 two, three, four bedroom units. Number of units for grandparent caregivers to be de-termined based on applications.	Pre-construction Break ground January 2005
Champlain Village/Church of Messiah Housing Corporation	Detroit, Michigan	11 rental townhomes, 16 apartments. First admissions for grandparents caring for a child with a disability.	Construction Plan to open late 2005
Diakon Lutheran Social Ministries	Baltimore, Maryland	Planned to replicate Boston Grandfamilies. Already servicing grandparent families.	Project suspended 1 year ago after exploring since the late 90's
Century Place Development now Heartland Housing	Chicago, Illinois	Planned to replicate Boston Grandfamilies.	Initial Project suspended by the county

Housing Authority and Buffalo Housing Authority are public housing facilities that have developed specific units just for grandparent caregivers. Casa Familia, Kinship Village, and Elizabeth's Place are units for grandparent caregivers within senior independent living facilities. Champlain Village is part of an urban revitalization project and is committed to having units specifically for grandparent caregivers.

Boston GrandFamilies House, Boston Housing Authority, Buffalo Housing Authority, and Casa Familia all currently have residents. PSS and Champlain Village are currently under construction and Elizabeth's Place and Kinship Village are in the pre-construction phase. Diakon Lutheran Social Ministries and Century Place Development (now Heartland Housing) have had their projects suspended due to operating obstacles.

Method: Representatives of the eight properties or development companies participated in a semi-structured telephone interview. Each interview lasted approximately 45 minutes. The interview (see Table 2) consisted of 11 semi-structured questions including: *What type of programs and services do you/or will you be providing to the (a) older adult and (b) the children?* and *What are the rules and regulations of the property (including the age and health requirements for both the older adult and child).* Extensive notes were taken during the interview. The majority of the questions were open ended, thereby allowing the participants to provide considerable detail. A cross comparative method was used to glean both basic descriptives about each site from the notes as well as key cross-cutting themes.

TABLE 2. Interview Questions for Grandparent Housing Programs

(1). What type of programs and services do you/or will you be providing to the (a) older adult and (b) the children?
(2). How are your individual housing units designed to accommodate older adults and children? (include size, furnishings, any specialized equipment, number of occupants allowed)
(3). What are the rules and regulations of the property? (include the age and health requirements for both older adult and child)
(4). Where do client referrals come from and what is the application process? (include wait list if any, cost of application)
(5). What are the qualifications of your staff, their training?
(6). What are the rules about the middle generation moving in? (parents of the child)
(7). What are the plans if a grandparent or relative caregiver dies or becomes ill while in residence?
(8). How is your program funded?
(9). What is the monthly cost for a family and how is this determined?

RESULTS

Services and Programs: All of the programs interviewed provided both generations of the families with services on site. Most of the staff had college degrees with backgrounds in social work, psychology, human services, education, and business. The facilities also utilized social work and early childhood interns. Some examples of programs for the grandparents in the housing programs includes support/education/information groups, grocery shopping, parenting workshops, field trips, bible study, nutrition programs, case management, English as a second language classes, homemaker/chore service, community gardens, and neighborhood watch groups. Several of the programs provided services to grandparents in collaboration with an on site senior center. As some of the programs were part of senior housing, senior center services, health clinics, and adult day care were also services available for the families. Local community agencies provide the day care services, for both children and adults.

The information provided to the grandparents in the support groups included legal assistance, long-term and financial planning, parenting skills, and health education. Connecting with the community was a key for many of the agencies to be able to provide comprehensive services for the families at a minimum expense. Several of the housing programs were enhancing existing services and therefore did not have to develop services specifically for caregiving grandparents.

Examples of services provided for children include after school, math/ science/computer learning centers, summer programs, youth employment, tutoring, and a homework helpline. The provision of day care services and after school programs was typically contracted to other agencies.

> One of the directors of the programs, Mrs. S, is also a grandparent caregiver and she lives on one of their properties. She states: The dynamics of families are changing and we need to figure out new ways to address it so these children can grow up whole. They (the children) come without clothes, shoes, and furniture. You have to figure out how to insure them and how to navigate the school system. It's very daunting, expensive. It cost me over $700 or $800 immediately and it was hard and I have a job. Most of these grandparents are living on subsidized income. How we expect them to make it? This housing program is wonderful.

Long-Term Plans: All of the programs reported that they had not considered the long-term health care needs of the caregiver prior to admission. In addition, none of the programs had realistic care plans for the children should the caregiver become hospitalized. The programs reported that they did have emergency numbers to contact should something happen to the grandparent.

Some of the programs reported that they wanted to have more programs and activities for teenagers.

Funding: Lack of funding was reported to be an obstacle to enhancing programs for the children. Both Boston and Buffalo Housing Authorities utilized Hope VI to fund the units developed for grandparent-headed households. Boston Grandfamilies, Presbyterian Social Services, Elizabeth's Place and Champlain Village all currently hold or are waiting for CHDO status. Casa Familia developed its program with state, city, and private funding mechanisms. Important elements of all of the housing programs were the community partnerships to provide ongoing services to the families.

Rules and Regulations of the Programs: There were several categories for rules and regulations of the housing programs. Most of the admissions regulations were related to the ages of the caregiver and care recipient, and the legal status of the caregiving relationship. Table 3 outlines the admissions rules and the financial obligations of the residents. All of the programs required that the primary caregiver be independent. Most of the facilities also allowed children to stay in the home after age 18 but they had to be enrolled in either college or a job training program. None of the facilities has yet to address what to do with an adult grandchild who is not in school. However, Boston Housing Authority does have a plan in place to relocate the grandparent to another home should a grandchild "age out" of the program.

With the exception of Elizabeth's Place and PSS, all of the programs require a formal legal custody relationship between the grandparents and grandchildren. Many of the families receive Section 8 vouchers to support their housing and therefore have to follow the regulations of that program. Although the Fair Housing Act prevents discrimination against grandparents with grandchildren, most properties wrote in custody or guardianship rules in their bylaws during construction phases prior to the first resident being admitted. Elizabeth Place's director explained why they have chosen not to require custody as part of admissions.

> Grandparents do not have to have formalized arrangements because the majority of the grandparents in this community do not have guardianship and they do not want to single anyone out, because this is part of the reason the grandparents are having difficulty obtaining housing in other places. We will not place a custody requirement, but social services will assist them with this matter. Long term planning will be encouraged not demanded.

None of the facilities would allow the children's parent to become a resident. Some reported that having the middle generation move in would defeat

TABLE 3. Housing Programs' Admission Rules and Funding

Facility Name/ Developer	Age Criteria	Legal Status	Funding
Boston Grandfamilies	Grandchildren–Must be under age 18. Can stay in housing until age 23 as long in college or vocational training. Grandparent– should be 50 plus	Permanent Legal custody	30% of income for rent Section 8 Will accept private pay Rent is between $700 and $800
Boston Housing Authority	Grandchildren–Must be between 6 and 17 years of age. Following High School graduation children must be in school or vocational program. Grandparent– any age but must be independent	Permanent Legal Custody	30% of income for rent Section 8 TANF funds Must be low income
Buffalo Housing Authority	Grandchildren–under age 18 at admission Grandpar-ent–any age but must be in-dependent	Permanent Legal Custody	30% of income for rent Section 8 TANF funds Must be low income HOPE VI grant
Casa Familia/ Casa Otonal	Grandchildren–Must be under 18 Grandparent–55 plus	Permanent Legal Custody	Section 8 Will accept private pay
Grandparent Family Apartments/ Presbyterian Social Services	Grandchildren–under 18 Grandparent–55 plus	No legal status necessary	Must be at or 50% below area's median income
Kinship Village/Fairhill Center for Aging	Not yet determined Pro-posed Grandchildren–under 18 Grandparent–55 plus	Not yet determined	Own formula based on income. Section 8
Elizabeth's Place/ Grandfamilies Housing Task Force	Grandchildren–under 18 Grandparent–no set age	No legal status necessary	Sliding Scale based on income Section 8 Will accept private pay
Champlain Village/Church of Messiah Housing Corporation	Grandchildren–under 18Grandparent–55 plus	Legal custody	Income under $28,000 Section 8 Rent $350-$700

the purpose of having the specialized housing. Since many of the grandparents were caring for their grandchildren due to parental substance abuse, allowing the parent in the home could also be a risk for the family and the community. One facility stated that they had a situation where the child's parent was found living in the grandparent home and using illegal substances. The family was consequently evicted. As one director stated

If they (child's parent) are living there illegally it usually becomes a problem and handled appropriately. The grandparents have difficulty setting limits. The families that they currently have most of the children's parents have passed away, others may visit periodically.

Occasionally emergencies occur where assistance with the child is needed.

If grandparent is ill or recently discharged from the hospital another adult may stay a few months after surgery, but usually this is an aunt or uncle and not the child's parent.

DISCUSSION AND RECOMMENDATIONS

Safe, affordable and accessible housing is an important consideration for grandparent caregiving families, the communities they live in, service providers, and policy makers. Interviews with staff at current and developing housing models suggest they are providing extraordinary comprehensive care for the grandparent-headed households they are serving. The abundance of services, support, and quality of housing also appear to greatly benefit the families in their residences. These families are less likely to fall through bureaucratic cracks. However, the need for development and operating funding was reported to be a significant barrier to the success of these housing programs. A national study of housing needs of grandparent caregivers as proposed by the LEGACY Act would add to the knowledge base of the needs for grandparents raising grandchildren.

Housing and the Other Critical Grandparent Issues. Illness, disease, and disability are problems that can strike anyone. Previous research has identified grandparent caregivers as being particularly vulnerable to physical, mental, and emotional impairments subsequent to becoming a caregiver. Existing and developing grandparent-housing programs need to consider the long-term care needs of both the grandparent caregivers and the children under their care. The interviews did not suggest that a lot of attention is being paid to these issues. Increased accessibility and ability to modify existing structures may help prevent any displacement of grandparent care should disability of the caregiver occur. In addition, strategies for having an alternate caregiver for the child on record were under-developed. By having a plan in place, the child would experience less disruption in his or her life and the grandparent caregiver can concentrate on getting well.

Status of the grandparent-grandchild relationship is another area that requires further exploration. Many grandparents have physical custody of their grandchildren rather than legal custody. Obtaining legal custody requires retaining a lawyer and taking time from work to go to court, an expense that many grandparents cannot afford. Additionally, many grandparents are reluctant to pursue a formal legal relationship with their grandchildren for fear of further straining their relationship with their own children (Fuller-Thomson & Minkler, 2003). The custody requirements of many programs limit access to services that would benefit their families. Rather than have a legal relationship as a requirement for admissions, more programs should consider admitting families regardless of the custody status (Fuller-Thomson & Minkler, 2003).

Future Directions. More model housing projects need to develop nationwide as a means of providing comprehensive services and resources to these families. Funding for the LEGACY Act would greatly enhance the ability of the existing and planned grandparent caregiver housing programs to provide services for grandparent-headed households. In particular, it would provide funding for HUD workers to receive training on the special needs of these households. In addition, funding needs to be available to grandparents who do not need to move but must expand or improve upon their existing homes as outlined in the LEGACY Act.

In the past few years more attention has been given to the unique needs of grandparent caregivers. Senator Clinton introduced the Kinship Caregiver Support Act on July 21st, 2004. This legislation would provide federal funding for development of service linkages for kinship caregivers as well as 4-E funding for relative caregivers. Another major piece of legislation that should benefit grandparent caregivers is The National Family Caregiver Support Act. This act permits 10% of its funding to be directed to assist older grandparents and other relatives raising children (Generations United, 2003). Across the nation, States are proposing and passing laws that acknowledge and provide assistance for grandparent caregivers. Some of these initiatives include subsidized guardianship, medical consent, and power of attorney for a minor child. While it is a great achievement that this population is finally getting recognition there is still much work to be done.

IMPLICATIONS FOR SOCIAL WORKERS

Long-term care planning and legal issues are two critical areas for grandparent families that affect housing options. Social workers need to educate families early in their caregiving process about obtaining legal custody of their grandchildren. In addition, having a clear plan in place for the children should the caregiver fall ill is vital to ensuring the least possible disruption for the family. Social workers also need to work with agencies to change policies regarding custody status. Grandparent families should be eligible to receive all services regardless of the legal status of the caregiving relationship. Agencies need to become sensitive to the unique family dynamics of grandparent-headed households and should not exclude families from receiving services based on lack of legal custody. The housing settings identified in this study may be ideal venues for the development of more grandparent caregiver friendly services.

Advocating to local, state, and federal legislators is necessary to ensure policy changes. On October 15, 2003 in Washington, DC, GrandRally was the first national gathering of grandparent families. This rally provided caregivers with the opportunity to have their voices heard by their representatives as well as uniting grandparent-headed families from across the country. This rally proved to be very successful. Families met others who were coping with similar issues and heard from important agencies that are working to make their lives better. Two months following this rally, the LEGACY Act was signed. Social workers concerned about housing for grandparent caregivers must become more active in lobbying policy makers to provide funding to make the proposals of the LEGACY Act a reality. In addition, social workers need to continue to empower families to advocate for themselves. Grandparents can communicate their experiences better than anyone else can. Again the housing programs identified may be ideal venues for educating grandparent families about advocacy.

CONCLUSION

Grandparent-headed households face enormous challenges. Grandparents should be rewarded for their hard work and for answering beyond the call of duty rather than be penalized for caring. To date limited housing options and financial assistance are harming rather than helping these families. Affordable and accessible housing should be a right rather than a privilege. Funding, education, and advocacy are crucial to helping these families provide safe homes for the children in their care.

REFERENCES

American Association of Retired Persons (AARP). (2004). *AARP: State Fact Sheets for Grandparents and Other Relatives Raising Children.* Retrieved May 6, 2004, from *http://research.aarp.org/general/kinship_care.html.*

Bloom, H. S., & Bloom, S. E. P. (1984). Household participation in the section 8 existing housing program. *Evaluation-Review. 5*(3), 325-40, 1981.

Burnette, D. (1997). Grandparents Raising Grandchildren in the Inner City. *Families in Society, 78*(5), 489-501.

Burnette, D. (1999). Custodial Grandparents in Latino Families: Patterns of Service Use and Predictors of Unmet Needs. *Social Work, 44*(1), 22-34.

Burton, L., & DeVries, C. (1992). Challenges and rewards: African American Grandparents as surrogate parents. *Generations, 16*(3), 51-54.

Casper, L., & Bryson, K. (1998). *Co-Resident Grandparents and Their Grandchildren: Grandparent Maintained Families.* Population Division U.S. Bureau of the Census Washington, DC.

Dalaker, J. (2001). *Poverty in the United States: 2000.* Washington, DC: US Government Printing Office.

Emick, M. A., & Hayslip, B. Jr. (1996). Custodial Grandparenting: New Roles for Middle Aged and Older Adults. *International Journal of Aging and Human Development, 43*(2), 135-154.

Emick, M. A., & Hayslip, B. (1999). Custodial grandparenting: Stresses, coping skills, and relationships with grandchildren. *International Journal of Aging and Human Development, 48*(1), 35-61.

Fuller-Thomson, E., & Minkler, M. (2003). Housing issues and realities facing grandparent caregivers who are renters. *The Gerontologist, 43*(1), 92-98.

Generations United (2003). Fact Sheet: Grandparents and others raising grandchildren: Their inclusion in the National Family Caregiver Support Program. Retrieved April 4, 2004 from *http://www.gu.org/Files/GuNFCSPFSNov03.pdf.*

Kanders, K. (2002). *Mind the gap: Grandparents raising grandchildren.* Retrieved May 5, 2004 from. *http://www.bos.frb.org/commdev/c&b/2002/spring/gf.pdf.*

Kolomer, S., McCallion, P., & Janicki, M. (2002). African-American Grandmother Carers of Children with Disabilities: Predictors of Depressive Symptoms. *Journal of Gerontological Social Work, 37*(3/4), 45.

Kolomer, S. R., & McCallion, P. (2005). Depression and Caregiver Mastery in grandfathers caring for their grandchildren. *International Journal of Aging and Human Development, 4*(60), 283-294.

Kornhaber, A. (1986). *Between parents and grandparents.* New York, NY: Martin's Press.

Minkler, M., Roe, K. M., & Price, M. (1992). The physical and emotional health of grandmothers raising grandchildren in the crack cocaine epidemic. *The Gerontologist, 32*(6), 752-761.

Minkler, M., & Roe, K. M. (1993) *Grandmothers as Caregivers: Raising children of the crack-cocaine epidemic.* Newbury Park, CA: Sage Publications, Inc.

Popkin, S. J., Katz, B., Cunningham, K. D., Brown, J., Gustafson, J., & Turner, M. A. (2004). *A decade of HOPE VI: Research finding and policy challenges.* Washington. DC: The Urban Institute and the Brookings.

Rental Housing Online (2005). Section 8 Rental Assistance Section 8 changed: Housing Choice Voucher Program. Retrieved May 12, 2005 from *http://cses.com/rental/section8.htm.*

Silverstein, N. M., & Vehvilainen, L. (1998). *Raising Awareness about Grandparents Raising Grandchildren in Massachusetts.* University of Massachusetts-Boston: Gerontology Institute.

Technical Assistance Program. (2005). Section 8 Housing Choice Voucher Program. Retreived May 11, 2005 from *http://www.tacinc.org/index/viewPage.cfm?pageId = 125.*

U.S. Census Bureau. (2002). American Community Survey Summary Tables. Grandparents Responsible for Own Grandchildren Under 18 Years by Sex of Grandparents in Households. In PCT014 (Ed.).

US Department of Housing and Urban Development–HUD (2005). Hope VI. Retreived May 5, 2005. *http://www.hud.gov/offices/pih/programs/ph/hope6/index.cfm.*

US Department of Housing and Urban Development–HUD (2005). CHDO Toolbox for HOME PJs. Retreived June 22, 2005. *http://www.hud.gov/offices/cpd/affordablehousing/library/modelguides/2004/200408.pdf.*

United States Department of Justice. Fair Housing Act. Section 802. 42 U.S.C. 3602 (k), Section 803. 3604 (b), (Supp.1994). Retreived June 22, 2005 *http://www.usdoj.gov/crt/housing/title8.htm.*

United States Department of Justice. Fair Housing Act. Section 807. 42 U.S.C. 3602 (k), Section 807. 3607 (b) 1, (Supp.1994). Retreived June 22, 2005 *http://www.usdoj.gov/crt/housing/title8.htm.*

doi:10.1300/J083v49n01_04

The Application of the Olmstead Decision on Housing and Eldercare

Elizabeth Palley, PhD, JD, MSW
Philip A. Rozario, PhD

SUMMARY. This article reviews the Supreme Court's interpretation of Title II of the Americans with Disabilities Act (ADA) and discusses its application for the frail older person. The parallels and differences between the societal ideas about, and the development of, community-based housing programs for younger populations of people with disabilities and for aging populations will be examined. This article explains how frail older people may be included in the ADA's definition of persons with disabilities. It then explains the Supreme Court's interpretation of discrimination in *Olmstead v. L.C. ex rel Zimring* (1999). Lastly, it examines the implications of the Olmstead decision for long-term care as it relates to housing for older people. doi:10.1300/J083v49n01_05 *[Article copies available for a fee from The Haworth Document Delivery Service: 1-800-HAWORTH. E-mail address: <docdelivery@haworthpress.com> Website: <http://www.HaworthPress.com> © 2007 by The Haworth Press, Inc. All rights reserved.]*

[Haworth co-indexing entry note]: "The Application of the Olmstead Decision on Housing and Eldercare." Palley, Elizabeth, and Philip A. Rozario, Co-published simultaneously in *Journal of Gerontological Social Work* (The Haworth Press, Inc.) Vol. 49, No. 1/2, 2007, pp. 81-96; and: *Housing for the Elderly: Policy and Practice Issues* (ed: Philip McCallion) The Haworth Press, Inc., 2007, pp. 81-96. Single or multiple copies of this article are available for a fee from The Haworth Document Delivery Service [1-800-HAWORTH, 9:00 a.m. - 5:00 p.m. (EST). E-mail address: docdelivery@haworthpress.com].

Available online at http://jgsw.haworthpress.com
© 2007 by The Haworth Press, Inc. All rights reserved.
doi:10.1300/J083v49n01_05

KEYWORDS. Housing, least restrictive environment, eldercare, long term care

INTRODUCTION

Social workers in the field of gerontology often deal with issues of elder care and housing. As a result, it is important for them to be informed about their clients' legal rights. Though older people with functional life skills limitations are not always perceived to be people with disabilities, many of the functional limitations of *frail* older people and persons with disabilities may be identical. If frail older people have sufficient limitations such that they are perceived to be people with disabilities, they may have additional civil rights afforded by the Americans with Disabilities Act (ADA). Among other things, these rights may protect older adults from unnecessary institutionalization and allow them to receive services in less restrictive settings.

In 1999, the Supreme Court of the United States held that unnecessary institutionalization of people with disabilities is discrimination and violates Title II of the ADA (*Olmstead v. L.C. ex. rel. Zimring*, 1999). Title II of the ADA states that a person with a disability cannot be discriminated against by a public entity (ADA, 2001). Because many older people, at some point in their lives, may fall within the ADA's definition of a person with a disability, this paper examines the implications of the Olmstead decision regarding long-term care for older citizens particularly related to housing issues.

This paper will examine circumstances in which elder care can be viewed as both a housing and a disability rights issue. It will then explain how federal laws and the Supreme Court have defined a person with a disability and how frail older people may fall into this definition. This discussion will be followed by an examination of the current state of the law regarding Title II of the ADA and the Olmstead decision. Lastly, this paper will discuss the current issues in the implementation of the Olmstead decision.

ELDER CARE AND DISABILITIES: ISSUES RELATED TO HOUSING

Although the need for long-term care services is evident across the lifespan, older adults account for a significantly higher proportion of people requiring long-term care services (Lucas, Schiller, & Benson, 2004; Robert Wood Johnson Foundation, 1996). Family and friends provide much of the care to their frail older relatives in the community under the rubric of long-term. However, for purposes of this paper, we are focusing on a group of older people who require the receipt of formal care services to meet their daily needs.

Long-term care cannot be easily defined because it includes both medical care and custodial elements (Aronson, 2002; Feldman & Kane, 2003). Kane (2001) defines long-term care as "personal care and assistance that an individual might receive on a long-term basis because of a disability or chronic illness that limits his or her ability to function" (p. 294). This definition disentangles long-term care services from the place where these services are provided. In addition, it is similar to the definition of disability under the ADA which states that someone is disabled if they are substantially limited in performing a major life activity (ADA, 1990). A key dimension of the long-term care service delivery involves the living arrangement of the person requiring assistance (Wilson, 1995).

Older adults with disabilities may sometimes have to decide on their housing options in the light of their reduced functional abilities. Oldman (2002) observes that both the location and suitability of living arrangements are important to people who are considered to be vulnerable. The majority of older people express their preference to live in their own homes for as long as they can (Gitlin, 2003). Thus, the ability to choose one's place of residence in order to receive long-term care services becomes an expression and exercise of one's freedom. Hawkins (1999) claims this is at the heart of human rights in old age. Although "older people generally hold varying, multiple, and potentially conflicting preferences for their LTC" (Kane & Kane, 2001, p. 114), social policies concerning housing and long-term care often fail to meet the wishes of older adults and their families in terms of their choice of residence when receiving long-term care. When older people are no longer able to compensate for their losses in the face of frailty, Steverink (2001) suggests that they might choose institutional care as a way to avoid further breakdown in their resources. Hence, the provision of formal home care would allow frail older people to continue living in their homes.

In order for older people with frailties to exercise their choice in living arrangement, we, as a society, need to make the necessary accommodations (Francis & Silvers, 2000). Pardeck (2001) argues that the passage of the Americans with Disabilities Act has important implications for health and human services policies and practices. To this end, older people with frailties can benefit from the gains that have been won by the disability rights' movement. Further as noted by Francis and Silvers, "the definition of disability . . . serves as a gatekeeping function in ADA jurisprudence: only the disabled can claim the statute's protection" (2000, p. 87).

Is the aim of care to ameliorate the disabling effects of frailty and chronic illnesses that the older person experiences or to slow the progression of the disabling conditions, or merely to feed and clothe the older person until he or she dies (Feldman & Kane, 2003)? The provision of long-term care in community settings may enable older people with frailties to continue to be a part of their community rather than to be merely sustained until death. As noted above, this follows from the philosophy of the disability rights' movement, the ADA, and the Olmstead decision. If elder care is defined as a disability rights' issue, older citizens who need life care assistance will be more likely to receive such assistance in a less restrictive environment.

SECTION 504 AND THE ADA

The federal government provided its first legislative protection for people with disabilities in 1973 when the Rehabilitation Act was passed. According to this law, "no otherwise qualified handicapped individual . . . shall, solely by reason of his/her handicap, be excluded from the participation in, be denied the benefits of, or be subject to discrimination under any program or activity receiving federal financial assistance" (Section 504 of the Rehabilitation Act, 1973). In 1990, these rights were expanded under the ADA to include protections against discrimination for people with disabilities by any agency that provides public services or employs 50 or more people. The ADA (1990) created an additional right for those who have been harmed to sue and receive monetary damages as well as attorney fees for instances in which they have been harmed as a result of an ADA violation.[1]

The ADA's (1990) goals are "to assure equality of opportunity, full participation, independent living, and economic self sufficiency," for people with disabilities assuming that this can be accomplished with "reasonable modifications" rather than the "fundamental alteration" of existing programs. The ADA includes several parts. When discussing issues of elder care and housing, Title II, part A is the most relevant section.

Title II part A provides that "no qualified individual with a disability shall, by reason of such disability, be excluded from participation in or be denied the benefits of the service, programs, or activities of a public entity, or be subjected to discrimination by any such entity" (ADA, 1990). A public entity is defined as "(A) any state or local government; (B) any department, agency, special purpose district (and) or other instrumentality of a State or States or local government" (ADA, 1990). This would therefore include any agency that acts on behalf of the state to provide long-term care and housing services to the frail older population.

Defining a Person with a Disability and Its Application to Elder Care

A person with a disability is defined as a person who:

  (i) has a physical or mental impairment which substantially limits one or more of such person's major life activities;
 (ii) has a record of such an impairment; or
(iii) is regarded as having such an impairment (ADA, 1990).

People are eligible for ADA (1990) protections if they either have a disability that "substantially limits one or more major life activities" or if they have "a record of such an impairment" or are "regarded as having such an impairment." Batavia (2001) notes that everyone in an institution getting services through Medicaid is arguably a person who is "regarded as" disabled even if the person does not actually require such services, because if a person was not perceived as disabled, he or she would not have institutional care paid for by Medicaid.

Some recent Supreme Court decisions have shed light on other aspects of the definition of a person with a disability. As noted above, the ADA requires that a person be "substantially limited" in their ability to perform "major life activities" in order to be protected by ADA civil right protections. Most of the cases in which the Supreme Court has sought to clarify these terms have addressed employment discrimination issues (Title I) rather than access to public services (Title II) (*Sutton v. United Airlines*, 1999; *Murphy v. U.S. Postal System*, 1999; *Albertson's v. Kirkingburg*, 1999; *Toyota v. Williams*, 2002). Nonetheless, the Supreme Court's guidance regarding a "substantial limitation" and a "major life activity" is relevant for Title II cases and, as such, must be understood when addressing issues of elder care and housing.

According to the Regulations to Implement the Equal Employment Provision of the ADA (1990) the term "substantially limits" means, "[u]nable to perform a major life activity that the average person in the general population can perform"; or "[s]ignificantly restricted as to the condition, manner or duration under which an individual can perform a particular major life activity as compared to the condition, manner, or duration under which the average person in the general population can perform that same major life activity." Further, "[m]ajor [l]ife [a]ctivities means functions such as caring for oneself, performing manual tasks, walking, seeing, hearing, speaking, breathing, learning, and working" (ADA, 1990).

The first case in which the Supreme Court assessed the meaning of "substantially limited" was *Sutton v. United Airlines* (1999). In this case, the Court held that "a person is taking measures to correct for, or mitigate, a physical or mental impairment, the effects of those measures–both positive and negative–must be taken into account when judging whether that person is 'substantially limited' in a major life activity and thus 'disabled' under the Act." They further noted, "To be sure, a person whose physical or mental impairment is corrected by mitigating measures still has an impairment, but if the impairment is corrected it does not 'substantially limi[t]' a major life activity" (*Sutton v. United Airlines*, 1999). This decision was supported by the decision in *Murphy v. U.S. Postal System* (1999).

The implication of these decisions for older people is reasonably clear. If an older person suffers from a disabling condition that has been ameliorated through medical care or assistive technology, the older person may not fall under the definition of disabled. If an older person is not considered to be disabled under the ADA, then the ADA will do nothing to ensure that the person can receive care in the least restrictive environment. Indeed, these cases raise some interesting questions for older people whose conditions might be ameliorated with assistive technology or medical care that they cannot afford and which is not covered by their insurance. Does someone merely need the theoretical capacity to have his/her condition ameliorated or must it actually be ameliorated? Some lower court decisions have suggested that if a person makes a conscious choice not to receive treatment for a treatable condition, then he or she would not be classified as disabled (*Tangires v. The Johns Hopkins Hospital*, 2000; *Spradley v. Custom Campers Inc.*, 1999).

The most recent case in which the Supreme Court addressed the issue of how to determine if someone is a person with a disability for purposes of ADA protections was *Toyota v. Williams* (2002). In this case, the Court found that the terms "substantial limitation" and "major life activity" "need to be interpreted strictly to create a demanding standard for qualifying as disabled." As a result, the court held "that to be substantially limited in performing manual tasks, an individual must have an impairment that prevents or severely restricts the individual from doing activities that are of central importance to most people's daily lives. The impairment's impact must also be permanent or long-term" (*Toyota v. Williams*, 2002, p. 197). This case was about a person who had carpal tunnel syndrome and could not perform factory line assembly functions.

However, this decision may have implications for elder care and housing. For example, if a patient has a broken hip and is expected to regain substantial amounts of his or her functional ability, depending upon the severity of the limitations which were caused by the break and the amount of ability the patient is expected to recover, the disabling condition might not be considered sufficient to allow the older person to be considered disabled for the purposes of the ADA and thus, not be eligible for federally-funded housing assistance nor be entitled to independent living assistance.

Though the Supreme Court has primarily addressed the definition of a disability as it relates to Title I, employment discrimination, the manner in which disability has been construed for purposes of Title I has implications for the entire ADA, including Title II. Still, despite the Supreme Court's guidance, there is no clear test as to how disabled a person must be in order to be protected by the ADA. The question remains: How do employment-related cases apply to the frail older population? The Supreme Court's interpretation of a person with a disability seems to suggest that if someone has a disabling or limiting condition that can be ameliorated with either personal compensatory skills (*Albertsons v. Kirkingburg,* 1999), assistive technology (*Sutton v. U.S. Airlines,* 1999), or medical care (*Murphy v. U.S. Postal System,* 1999), this person would not fall within the ADA's definition of a person with a disability. Because one must first be considered a person with a disability in order to be eligible for ADA protections, these cases are relevant to understand the extent of the ADA's protections for frail older people and the extent to which frail elders entitlement to independent living assistance is protected under the ADA.

THE OLMSTEAD DECISION AND ITS APPLICATION

In 1999, the Supreme Court held that the State of Georgia had violated Title II of the ADA by requiring two psychiatric patients to remain in a psychiatric hospital despite their medical providers' beliefs that these individuals could be served in a less restrictive environment. Though the State of Georgia provided services to similarly situated individuals in community-based settings, the two women in this case were forced to remain in a restrictive hospital setting because there were no spaces available in less restrictive community-based settings (*Olmstead v. L.C. ex rel. Zimring,* 1999).

The Olmstead decision created a standard for determining when states were in violation of Title II of the ADA. The Court held that the ADA does not require states to "fundamentally alter" their existing programs. States may calculate the cost of providing such services to persons with disabilities and balance these costs with the provision of other services that they are required to provide to others to decide if such services can be considered "fundamental alterations" to their existing programs. The Court directed states to "tak[e] into account the resources available to the state and the needs of others with mental disabilities" (*Olmstead v. L.C. ex rel. Zimring,* 1999).

In response to the Olmstead decision in January of 2000, Donna Shalala, the then Secretary of Health and Human Services, sent a cover letter to governors including a guidance letter authored by Timothy Westmoreland, Director of the Center for Medicaid and State Operations for Health Care Financing

Administration, and Thomas Perez, the Director of the Office of Civil Rights, which was originally written for state Medicaid directors suggesting that states could comply with the ADA "by having comprehensive, effectively working plans ensuring that individuals with disabilities receive services in the most integrated setting appropriate to their needs" (Westmoreland & Perez, 2000). In other words, if states have plans, it may be acceptable to have wait lists that move at a reasonable pace.

The 9th Circuit is the only circuit to address the provision of care specifically for an older adult. In this case, Levi Townsend claimed that Washington State's Medicaid policy, in which "medically needy" and "categorically needy" are able to receive different levels of care, violated his ADA integration mandate. The 9th Circuit remanded the case to the district court with the direction that "the denial of community-based long-term care for "medically needy" disabled persons violates the ADA unless the Secretary can demonstrate that extending eligibility to these persons would fundamentally alter its Medicaid program" (*Townsend v. Quasim, 2003*).

Several lower court decisions have followed with their own interpretations of the Olmstead decision, particularly regarding what a "fundamental alteration" is and on these grounds, whether states have discriminated against people with disabilities. These cases provide some insight into the factors that courts will consider. For example, in *Rodriguez v. City of New York* (1999), the Second Circuit found that creating a new Medicaid service to ensure safety monitoring which would allow people with mental disabilities to live in the community would be a "fundamental alteration" of the existing program and therefore, was not required. In a Pennsylvania case, where institutionalized mentally ill adults who were seeking community-based placement and found eligible for such placement, the Third Circuit held that the Department of Public Welfare's decision not to increase community-based placements was consistent with Olmstead because, based on the Department's fiscal analysis, an increase in placements would require a "fundamental alteration" in services to other people receiving services through the Department (*Frederick L. v. Department of Public Welfare of Pennslyvania*, 2004).

In a recent 10th Circuit case, the court held that an Oklahoma community-based Medicaid waiver program that placed a five prescription cap on community living recipients and not on nursing home residents was discriminatory, and would likely be more expensive for the state as some people would be unable to remain in the community with such caps and be forced to go to nursing homes where their care would cost more. Further the court noted that "Olmstead rejected a construction of the fundamental alteration defense that required only a comparison of the cost of community services for the plaintiffs with the state's budget" (*Katherine Fisher v. Oklahoma Health Care Authority,* 2003).

Moreover, the Hawaii District Court found that Title II does not allow waiver programs to be capped even though Medicaid would allow such caps. The Court found that this was not a "fundamental alteration" of the Medicaid waiver program. In this case, the Court found that Hawaii had discriminated against people with mental retardation by not having a comprehensive plan to get them off wait lists and into community settings (*Makin v. Hawaii*, 1999). As a result, they were required to alter their program to reduce the number of people with mental retardation in institutional facilities and move them into community settings.

In a Maryland District Court case (*Williams v. Wasserman,* 2001), the court found that, based on the Olmstead test, though it might ultimately be cheaper to provide services to people with disabilities in the community, it would not immediately be less expensive since the cost of the institutional care would remain the same while additional costs were incurred by some people who received community-based services. The court held that Maryland had a history of moving people into community-based settings and on those grounds; they should be able to gradually change their services in order not to have to incur undue expenses.

The lower courts seem to be sending different messages regarding the extent to which costs may be considered when states make long-term care decisions for people with disabilities. Only four Circuit courts have addressed the issue of implementing the Olmstead requirements in regards to community-based placements. Three of these have found that, because of the costs associated with increasing community-based placements or altering current policy to make community services easier to access, it would require "fundamental alterations" to existing programs; in those cases, states were not forced to provide less restrictive placements to plaintiffs. In Maryland, though, the court agreed that in the long term, community-based care would be less expensive and that, in the given cases, it might be more appropriate if the court allowed the state to win on a "fundamental alteration" and an expense-based argument. On the other hand, the Hawaii District Court required the State of Hawaii to significantly alter their services and create new services in order to comply with the Olmstead decision. For now, it seems that the state or district in which a person with a disability, including an older citizen, lives may alter the likelihood that he or she will be able to access care in the least restrictive environment.

ISSUES IN IMPLEMENTING THE OLMSTEAD DECISION IN LONG-TERM CARE PROGRAMS FOR OLDER PEOPLE

Funding issues and provider attitudes are key obstacles to the implementation of the ADA's least restrictive environment mandate. As noted above, according to the decision in Olmstead (1999), "the proscription of discrimination may require placement of persons with mental disabilities in community settings rather than institutions." The catch is the extent to which such systems of care already exist in a given state. The primary source of payment for such care is Medicaid (Miller, 2002). As a result, though Olmstead never mentions Medicaid, it is important to understand the implications of Medicaid policies for its implementation.

As noted by Rosenbaum, Teitelbaum, and Stewart (2002), "because the integration of persons with disabilities into the community depends so heavily on how States approach Medicaid financing, discussions about Olmstead quickly become discussions on Medicaid" (p. 94). Even when finances are not at issue, provider attitudes may create a barrier to the implementation of community-based care for frail older adults. Often these two obstacles operate in concert with each other to reduce the possibilities of community-based care for the older adults. This section of the paper will address both issues and identify some possible solutions.

Funding Issues

The confluence of increase in state expenditure on long-term care, decreased levels of federal funding and other state revenues, and the political and ideological shifts in the provision of publicly-funded services has threatened the implementation of the Olmstead decision (Aronson, 2002; Weil, 2003). Indeed, Li and Zullo (2003) reported that Michigan suspended its enrollment into the Michigan Choice program because of budgetary constraints in 2001. Further, the lack of clarity as to what constitutes "reasonable accommodations," as specified in Title II of the ADA, may complicate the implementation of the Olmstead decision in the face of higher levels of need.

While home care is often considered a cheaper alternative to premature institutional care, there are many reasons that might prevent the immediate implementation of the Olmstead decision in providing care in the least restrictive environment. At the state programmatic level, the Maryland District Court ruled that the state might not need to aggressively implement the Olmstead decision if the cost of implementing the community-based program is too expensive for the state to bear. On the individual level, the cost of home care can become prohibitive when the person requires care and supervision on a 24-hour basis. In such instances, the frail older person may no longer be reasonably accommodated within the community.

Medicaid and Medicaid Waiver

Medicaid is a health insurance program for low-income people, including those who are categorized as older and disabled. Since it was originally enacted, the program has expanded to cover low-income single mothers and their children, as well as certain low-income older people who are eligible for assistance with Medicare cost-sharing (Weil, 2003). Medicaid requires that the services it provides, "(i) shall not be less in amount, duration, or scope than the medical assistance made available to any other such individual, and (ii) shall not be less in amount, duration, or scope than the medical assistance made available to individuals . . ." (Medicaid, Grants to States for Medical Assistance Programs, 42 USC § 1396a, 1998). Further, special provisions are made for people who are eligible for institutional and home-based waiver services even if their income levels exceed the supplemental security income (SSI) levels (Bruen, Wiener, Kim, & Miazad, 1999). In 1998, Medicaid funded about 39% of long-term care in the U.S., the majority of which was spent on nursing home and intermediate care facilities for the mentally retarded (Miller, 2002). Weil (2003) argues that Medicaid is best-suited to meet the challenges of a new health policy (including the Olmstead decision) because its existing infrastructure is flexible enough to respond to the changing needs of the public.

Long before the Olmstead decision, the Medicaid Waiver program was instituted to provide community-based long-term care services to those who would otherwise receive such services in an institutional setting. The Medicaid Waiver Program has a number of positive features in that it allows states some flexibility in deciding the scope, type, and amount of services in each state (Weil, 2003). Further, each state can set the income and resources eligibility guidelines for their long-term care services under the Medicaid waiver program (Bruen, Wiener, Kim, & Miazad, 1999). Weil (2003) argues that "Medicaid has become the workhorse of the U.S. health care system because the program has been used to meet the health and long-term care needs of various groups in the population" (p. 15). The flexibility inherent in the waiver programs represents a double-edged sword, in that some states can decide on providing the minimum in their scope, type, and amount of services or instituting stricter levels of eligibility criteria. As such, Weil (2003) recommends a statutory revision of the waiver program that would allow states to simplify their eligibility and provisions.

Morgan and David (2002) argue that the Medicaid system is currently set up for older people to lose because in order to qualify for publicly-funded services they need to have limited assets and income or to spend down their financial resources. With such limited resources, they may be unable to remain in the community. Further, it is not always clear that the older person will be eligible for community-based care as they spend down their resources in hopes of accessing appropriate services when they are needed. Unlike the two women in the Olmstead case, an older person may not have time left in their life to challenge a state's decision regarding their care in a court case. The statutory provisions should include expedited processing of applications and appeals where older people in greatest need of publicly-provided long-term care services are not left waiting for long periods before finding out about their eligibility.

Providers' Attitudes

As mentioned earlier, the success of the implementation of the Olmstead decision's preference for long-term care services in the least restrictive environment lies in part with the attitudes that service providers have with regard to frail older persons. These attitudes may stem from different philosophical orientations of the disability and aging movements. The underlying philosophy of the disability movement is more likely to emphasize consumer choice, while that of the aging movement is more likely to underscore the management of care on behalf the individual (Putnam, 2002). Interestingly, while younger people with disabilities have moved out from institutional care to community settings, "policy makers and service providers continue to regard institutional care as a legitimate form of care for older people" (Walker, Walker, & Gosling, 1999, p. 116). Indeed some even question whether or not older people want the responsibilities of managing their own care services and whether they are capable of undertaking such responsibilities (Tilly & Wiener, 2001). This often results in the imposition of restrictions on their options and opportunities for the receipt of publicly-funded housing services when they have long-term care needs.

Care providers' paternalistic attitudes may prevent older people from taking negotiated risks, and this can potentially harm the psychological well-being of older people and limit their ability to live in less restrictive settings. Indeed, older people in need of long-term care services might be reluctant to express those needs to their care providers for fear that they may be placed in a nursing home. For example, in her qualitative study on older women receiving home care, Aronson (2002) found that some of the respondents reported that they had to be circumspect and self-protective with their case managers so as to avoid being labeled "nursing home material" (p. 405). Kane and Kane (2001) assert that this attitude and these practices may stem from our ageist notions about older people. As such it is important for social workers to discuss long-term care and housing options with older clients, as well as their family members, with the view of emphasizing the clients' sense of autonomy and independence.

Appropriate Placements

Frail older individuals have different levels of functioning–as measured by their ability to perform activities of daily living and instrumental activities of daily living–and needs. Further, unlike other populations of people with disabilities, the health status of a frail older person is subject to constant change. While frail older people may require help in performing some of the activities of daily living, we need to ensure that we maintain their functional competence so as to enhance their quality of life (Kane, 2001). Feldman and Kane (2003) report research findings that show improvements in frail older people's functioning when staff had higher expectations of their care recipients.

These studies reviewed by Feldman and Kane (2003) suggest that systems of care should be developed for older people that enable them to easily transition between home and community-based care to more restrictive settings as necessary. This requires the availability and affordability of both appropriate services for both long-term care services and housing. This cannot be accomplished with Medicaid's current requirements that people spend down their assets in order to be eligible for housing assistance. If people spend down their assets, they will be unable to afford to move back into the community from a nursing facility should such a move be possible. In addition, the "spend down" requirements make it impossible for older adults to be able to access most community-based services until they are indigent and must be placed in a nursing facility. For social workers in the field of gerontology, this means conducting regular assessments and updated plans so that their long-term care clients are appropriately placed in suitable environments according to their needs and abilities.

CONCLUSIONS

According to the Olmstead decision, states may be found to be in violation of the ADA if the state provides community-based care and does not make it available to the disabled, including, but not limited to, older disabled citizens who can live in a less restrictive setting with appropriate support services. Though 39% of all community-based and residential care services are paid for by Medicaid funds, the Olmstead decision does not mention Medicaid. In addition, the Olmstead decision specifically notes that states may balance the care that is provided to one person against the system of care for all (*Olmstead v. L.C. ex. Rel Zimring*, 1999). Further, the ADA only requires reasonable modifications rather than a major restructuring of care systems in order to be in compliance. If a state has no community-based options available for anyone, then, despite the fact that such care may be less restrictive for an older person, the state may not be required to provide such care.

The implications of the Olmstead decision for long-term care and housing for frail older people are less than clear. The existence of state community-based care systems will influence the extent to which Olmstead will encourage the expansion of such care. If these systems do not already exist, states must work toward providing less restrictive services but the speed at which they must change their services is less clear. In addition, if states can demonstrate that the cost of such changes would affect the care for others who are similarly situated, it is possible that they may be able to continue to use restrictive care settings. Nonetheless, Olmstead does specifically note that states may be violating their citizens' rights by maintaining them in facilities that are more restrictive than they need to be. If people can be placed in less restrictive settings without burdensome costs to the states, states will likely be required to provide more community-based services. Further, because systems of care for older citizens have often been created using provider attitudes that limit the control that older people can have on their own care decisions, they often receive care in settings that are more restrictive than they need to be.

These systems may also be more expensive than some home-based care. The literature suggests that a range of care and flexibility for older citizens to move between levels of care with relative ease may be both the most appropriate and most fiscally achievable policy. In this article, we suggest that expansions and clarification of Medicaid Waiver programs could help facilitate these changes. However, at present, though the ADA suggests a preference toward providing care in less restrictive settings, all older citizens may not be provided with these options as a matter of law.

NOTE

1. The Supreme Court has since held that the right to receive monetary damages for state violations of Title I is unconstitutional (*Garrett v. University of Alabama*, 2001). Because the issue which this article discusses does not address the issue of financial remuneration for injuries which are caused by violations of the ADA, the application of this Title I case will not be discussed in this article.

REFERENCES

Albertson's v. Kirkingburg, 527 U.S. 555 (1999).
Americans with Disabilities Act (1990). 42 USC § 12100 et. seq.
Aronson, J. (2002). Elderly people's accounts of home care rationing: Missing voices in long-term care policy debates. *Ageing and Society, 22,* 399-418.
Batavia, A. I. (2002). A right to personal assistance services: "Most integrated setting appropriate" requirements and the Independent Living Model of long term care. *American Journal of Law and Medicine, 27,* 17-42.

Bruen, B. K., Wiener, J. M., Kim, J., & Miazad, O. (1999). *State usage of Medicaid coverage options for aged, blind, and disabled people.* Washington, DC: Urban Institute.

Feldman, P. H., & Kane, R. L. (2003). Strengthening research to improve the practice and management of long-term care. *The Milbank Quarterly, 81*(2), 179-220.

Fisher v. Oklahoma Health Care Authority, 335 F3d. 1175 (2003).

Francis, L., & Silvers, A. (2000). Achieving the right to live in the world: Americans with disabilities and the civil rights tradition. In L. Francis & A. Silvers (Eds.), *Americans with Disabilities: Implications for Individuals and Institutions* (pp. xiii-xxx). London: Routledge Press.

Frederick L. v. Department of Public Welfare of Pennslyvania, 364 F.3d 487 (2004).

Garrett v. University of Alabama, 531 U.S. 356 (2001).

Gitlin, L. N. (2003). Conducting research on home environments: Lessons learned and new directions. *The Gerontologist, 43*(5), 628-637.

Hawkins, B. A. (1999). Rights, place of residence, and retirement: Lessons from case studies on aging. In S. S. Herr & G. Weber (1999). *Aging, rights and quality of life: Prospects for older people with developmental disabilities* (pp. 93-107). Baltimore: Paul H. Brookes Publishing Company.

Kane, R. A. (2001). Long-term care and a good quality of life: Bringing them closer together. *The Gerontologist, 41*(3), 293-304.

Kane, R. L., & Kane, R. A. (2001). What older people want from long-term care, and how they can get it. *Health Affairs, 20*(6), 114-127.

Katherine Fisher v. Oklahoma Health Care Authority, 335 F.3d 1175 (2003).

Li, L., & Zullo, R. (2003). A functioning profile of Medicaid waiver participants in Michigan: Does the program admit the high functioning? *Care Management Journals, 4*(1), 31-36.

Lucas, J. W., Schiller, J. S., & Benson, V. (2004). Summary health statistics for US adults: National Health Interview Survey 2001. *National Center for Health Statistics–Vital Health Statistics, 10*(218).

Makin v. Hawaii, 114 F. Supp. 2d 1017 (D. Haw. 1999).

Medicaid, Grants to States for Medical Assistance Programs, 42 U.S.C. § 1396a. (1998).

Miller, E. A. (2002). State discretion and Medicaid program variation in long-term care: When is enough, enough? In G. G. Caro & R. Morris (Eds.), *Devolution and aging policy* (pp. 15-35). New York: The Haworth Press.

Morgan, R. E., & David, S. (2002). Human rights: A new language for aging advocacy. *The Gerontologist, 42*(4), 436-442.

Murphy v. U.S. Postal System, 527 U.S. 516 (1999).

Nondiscrimination on the Basis of Disability in State and Local Government Services (1992). 34 CFR Part 35.

Oldman, C. (2002). The importance of housing and home. In B. Bytheway, V. Bacigalupo, J. Bornat, J. Johnson, & S. Spurr (Eds.), *Understanding care, welfare, and community: A reader* (pp. 330-340). London: Routledge.

Olmstead v. L. C. by Zimring, 527 U.S. 581 (1999).

Pardeck, J. T. (2001). An update on the Americans with Disabilities Act: Implications for health and human service delivery. *Journal of Health & Social Policy, 13*(4), 1-15.

Putnam, M. (2002). Linking aging theory and disability models: Increasing the potential to explore aging with physical impairment. *The Gerontologist, 42*(6), 799-806.

Rehabilitation Act of 1973, 29 USC § 701 et. seq.

Robert Wood Johnson Foundation (1996). *Chronic care in America: A 21st century challenge.* Princeton: Author.

Rodriguez v. City of New York, 197 F 3d 611 (2nd Cir 1999), cert denied 121 SCT 156 (2000).

Rosenbaum, S., Teitelbaum, J., & Stewart, A. (2002). Symposium: Barriers to access to health care: *Olmstead v. L.C.*: Implications for Medicaid and other publically funded health services. *Case Western Reserve Health Matrix, Journal of Law-Medicine, 12,* 93-138.

Shalala, D. (2000), Secretary's letter to governors on Olmstead decision, January 14. Health Care Finance Administration. Retrieved on July 27, 2004 at *www.hcfa.gov/states/letters/smd1140b.htm.*

Spradley v. Custom Campers Inc., 68 F. Supp. 2d 1225 (D Kansas, 1999).

Steverink, N. (2001). When and why frail elderly people give up independent living: The Netherlands as an example. *Ageing and Society, 21,* 45-69.

Sutton v. United Airlines, 527 U.S. 471 (1999).

Tangires v. The Johns Hopkins Hospital, 79 F. Supp. 2d 587 (D MD, 2000).

Tilly, J., & Wiener, J. M. (2001). *Consumer-directed home and community services: Policy issues.* Occasional Paper 44. Washington, DC: The Urban Institute.

Townsend v. Quasim, 328 F.3d 511, 520 (2003).

Toyota v. Williams, 534 U.S. 184 (2002).

Walker, A., Walker, C., & Gosling, V. (1999). Quality of life as a matter of human rights. In S. S. Herr & G. Weber (1999). Aging, rights and quality of life: Prospects for older people with developmental disabilities (pp. 109-132). Baltimore: Paul H. Brookes Publishing Company.

Weil, A. (2003). There's something about Medicaid. *Health Affairs, 22*(1), 13-30.

Westmoreland, T. & Perez, T. (2000, January 14). Letter from the Health Care Finance Administration to State and the Office of Civil Rights to Medicaid Directors to provide guidance on the Olmstead Decision. Retrieved on May 12, 2005 at *http://www.cms.hhs.gov/states/letters/smd1140a.asp.*

Williams v. Wasserman, 164 F.Supp.2d 591 (D.Md. 2001)

Wilson, N. L. (1995) Long-term care in the United States: An overview of the current system. In L.B. McCullough & N.L. Wilson (Eds.), *Long-term care decisions: Ethical and conceptual dimensions* (pp. 35-59). Baltimore: Johns Hopkins University Press.

doi:10.1300/J083v49n01_05

Impact of the Olmstead Decision
Five Years Later:
A National Perspective for Social Workers

Anna L. Zendell, MSW

SUMMARY. The Olmstead Decision of 1999 continues to have the potential to radically transform the long-term care system in the United States. This article will review the components of the decision and steps being taken by the federal and state governments to address its challenges and mandates. A number of key areas where social workers can play important roles will be described. doi:10.1300/J083v49n01_06 *[Article copies available for a fee from The Haworth Document Delivery Service: 1-800-HAWORTH. E-mail address: <docdelivery@haworthpress.com> Website: <http://www.HaworthPress.com> © 2007 by The Haworth Press, Inc. All rights reserved.]*

KEYWORDS. Olmstead decision, long-term care, disabilities, social work roles, community integration

THE OLMSTEAD DECISION

Olmstead v. L.C. ex rel. Zimring represents a landmark judicial interpretation of the Americans with Disabilities Act (ADA) by the United States Supreme

[Haworth co-indexing entry note]: "Impact of the Olmstead Decision Five Years Later: A National Perspective for Social Workers." Zendell, Anna L. Co-published simultaneously in *Journal of Gerontological Social Work* (The Haworth Press, Inc.) Vol. 49, No. 1/2, 2007, pp. 97-113; and: *Housing for the Elderly: Policy and Practice Issues* (ed: Philip McCallion) The Haworth Press, Inc., 2007, pp. 97-113. Single or multiple copies of this article are available for a fee from The Haworth Document Delivery Service [1-800-HAWORTH, 9:00 a.m. - 5:00 p.m. (EST). E-mail address: docdelivery@haworthpress.com].

Court. The case was brought on behalf of two women dually diagnosed with mental retardation and mental illness. They were voluntary psychiatric patients confined to Georgia state psychiatric centers for over two years at the time the lawsuit was initiated in 1997. After a year or more of inpatient treatment, their professional treatment teams had determined that both women could be appropriately and safely served in a community setting (Bazelon, n.d.a.; Bazelon, n.d.b.; Smith & Calandrillo, 2001). Despite this determination, the two women remained institutionalized.

The plaintiffs claimed that Georgia was violating Title II of the ADA by failing to provide treatment in the community after it was deemed appropriate. Title II says "no qualified individual with a disability shall, by reason of such disability, be excluded from participation in, or denied benefits of, services, programs, or activities of a public entity, or be subjected to discrimination by any such entity" (Mathis, 2001, p. 395). The state argued that the ADA pertains only to the treatment of individuals with disabilities *as compared to* the treatment of individuals without a disability. It would not apply to people with disabilities who are receiving public services designed exclusively for their needs.

However, the Supreme Court determined that the continued institutionalization of these women constituted discrimination, or unnecessary segregation, and that people with disabilities have the right to live in the most integrated setting appropriate for their needs. Several justices compared the unjustifiable isolation of individuals with disabilities to racial discrimination and segregation. Their decision requires states that offer funding for–or actual–treatment or services to persons with disabilities to provide such services in the most integrated community setting appropriate (Legal Information Institute [LII], 1999; Smith & Calandrillo, 2001).

The Olmstead Decision applies to all individuals with disabilities, regardless of disability type, age, socioeconomic status, and ethnicity. It applies to any individual diagnosed with a physical or mental disability who is either at risk of being institutionalized due to lack of available community supports, or is institutionalized but could live in the community if resources were available. It may affect individuals with disabilities living in nursing homes, psychiatric hospitals, adult homes, jails and prisons, large and small community residences, children living in residential treatment facilities, the elderly, and those in other institutional settings (Bazelon, n.d.a; Cohen, 2001; Coleman, 2002; HHS, 2003a; Kafka, 2002; LII, 1999; Mathis; 2001; NAPAS, 2002; NAPAS, 2003; NCSL, n.d.; Rosenbaum & Teitelbam, 2004; Smith & Calandrillo, 2001).

The Olmstead decision set forth three circumstances which would allow states to disregard this requirement: (1) fundamental alteration due to cost, (2) destabilization of the existing service delivery system, and (3) individual preference (LII, 1999). First, the decision held that states are not required to provide community placement if the cost would represent a fundamental alteration in the state's programs. Fundamental alteration is defined as a change in the essential nature of the program, thereby imposing undue hardship on the state (ibid.). Community placements are not required if they would prevent states from maintaining a range of facilities to meet the widest range of needs and distribute services in an equitable manner for all persons with disabilities (Bazelon, n.d.a; LII, 1999; Smith & Calandrillo, 2001). Olmstead-related legislation, such as *Barthelemy et al. v. Louisiana Department of Health and Hospitals,* illustrates that cost of providing existing services to deinstitutionalized persons is not an adequate defense. In *Barthelemy v. Louisiana,* five institutionalized individuals sued the state of Louisiana for inappropriately restricting them to a nursing facility when services were available in the community in the form of nursing and home health care. The state ultimately settled the case, reaching an agreement to expand funding for home-based services over a period of four years in a manner that would not create fundamental alterations due to increased costs (Smith, 2002).[1]

Second, the most integrated setting would not be required if the result is a rapid shift of resources to community placements from nursing homes and psychiatric centers likely to cause destabilization of the institutional infrastructure (Bazelon, n.d.a; Bazelon, n.d.b; LII, 1999; Smith & Calandrillo, 2001). An example of Olmstead-related litigation on this point involves *Frederic I. v. Department of Public Welfare in Pennsylvania* in 2002, where plaintiffs represented residents at Norristown State Hospital denied community placement, despite expert recommendations of preparedness for community living. While the US Court of Appeals ruled that patients' rights were being violated, justices further ruled that expedited community placement would likely create increased expenditures and might decrease services available to other individuals in the state. The combined risks of increased expenditures and decreased services to others with disabilities led to a court decision in this matter that community placement would result in a probable fundamental alteration to the service delivery system (Smith, 2002). This fundamental alteration could also destabilize the balance between institutions and community-based services. States are exempted from offering community placement only if no funding is available to create such placements and no options to create funding exist. States using such a rationale must prove that no other funding sources exist.

Third, states are exempted from provision of community placement in the most integrated setting if beneficiaries do not want it (Bazelon, n.d.a; LII, 1999; Smith & Calandrillo, 2001). For example, some older adults prefer nursing homes or assisted living facilities over independent living for the increased opportunities for socialization. The same is true for some individuals with developmental, psychiatric, and physical disabilities who may have felt isolated in their homes in the community or who may fear the unknown of an independent living arrangement (Cohen, 2001).

NATIONAL IMPLEMENTATION OF THE OLMSTEAD DECISION

As a nation, the United States has experienced a slow start in implementing Olmstead. The Supreme Court did not specify compliance deadlines when the decision was rendered in 1999. Consequently, states differ tremendously in what they have accomplished in the years since the decision. The first step most states have taken is to set up Olmstead task forces, which, although not a mandate, have been strongly suggested by the White House (White House, 2001). As of December 2002, 43 states had initiated Olmstead task forces. Twenty-nine states had developed comprehensive Olmstead Plans or Reports as of June 2004.

A number of states have publicly stated they do not intend to create an Olmstead comprehensive plan, but are working on state-wide projects related to implementing the intent of the Olmstead Decision. Several states (Missouri, Nebraska, Montana, and Michigan) have established central offices to assist in plan formulation and implementation. Texas and Missouri have proposed changes to allow individuals' funding to follow them from institution to community settings. Twenty states have implemented Medicaid buy-in programs to allow people with disabilities at risk of losing their Medicaid insurance (due to obtaining employment or salary increase) to pay partial Medicaid premiums and retain their insurance. Alabama, Oregon, Ohio, and Massachusetts are exploring Olmstead-dedicated allocation of HUD Section 8 housing vouchers for people with disabilities. Another Olmstead-related initiative undertaken by several states is consumer-directed caregiver compensation, in which consumers can pay certain non-immediate family member caregivers to provide services (NAPAS, 2002 & 2003; National Conference of State Legislatures [NCSL], n.d.; Rosenbaum & Teitelbaum, 2004).

SOCIAL WORKER ROLES

Social workers can play pivotal roles in both policy implementation and advocacy for persons with disabilities. These include (1) interpreting the Olmstead decision through the political process, (2) attaining true integration of services, (3) reducing fragmentation of services, (4) transitioning people from institutions into the community, (5) assuring funding for individuals during transitions, (6) creating assessment tools, (7) addressing workforce issues, (8) balancing community and institutions, (9) promoting quality, (10) forging collaboration, (11) securing state-level funding, and (12) engaging in public advocacy.

(1) Interpreting the Decision

What is the *fundamental alteration* of services? What constitutes the *most integrated setting*? How do states define *reasonable pace* in resolving waiting lists? Although HHS has issued guidance letters, these key phrases are being operationally defined in different ways across the United States. Who is capable of benefiting from the most integrated setting and which wait lists should be addressed first are value based decisions. It is incumbent upon social workers to influence how states operationalize these phrases, utilizing their professional skills to clarify values and construct meaningful definitions. Social workers can bring to this task their knowledge of current service needs, the existing service delivery system, and service usage patterns. As key players in the service system, social workers can play a pivotal role in informing policy makers about court-imposed time limits, and how best to structure an effective plan.

Much of the general public appears to hold the view that the long-term care situation is acceptable, if not ideal, for most individuals with disabilities. In general, there is complacency with nursing homes, hospitals, and large community residences, even among many social work professionals. Social workers have become acculturated to these environments. Educating social workers about new opportunities for community integration and community-based services for persons institutionalized, in group homes, or at risk of such placements will be important in realizing the intent of Olmstead (Bartels et al., 2003). There are also public stereotypes, fears, and prejudices with which to contend. The past few years have revealed negative media attention about people with mental illness and in many cases framed them as a danger to the community. As a result, many communities do not want community residences for persons with disabilities in their neighborhoods. The notion of *not in my backyard* must be overcome before implementation can be successful. Implementation may also be hindered by conflicts between the elderly, children's advocates, and the adult disabilities communities, including those based on mental health, developmental disabilities, and physical disabilities (Coalition, 2003).

(2) Attaining True Community Integration

Ironically, large-scale community integration efforts can easily lead to a different type of segregation for people with disabilities (Donlin, 2003). People with disabilities and the elderly may end up in the community, but in segregated settings such as large apartment buildings, complexes, or houses specifically for people with disabilities, that deprive them of the *normal* community experiences of people without disabilities (Coalition, 2003). Some of this may be by ·choice. Some older people enjoy living in senior complexes where they have access to on-site services, transportation, and companionship they may not have access to living in more integrated communities. Likewise, some persons with disabilities prefer living in larger residential settings that provide greater activity and opportunity for companionship. Often persons with disabilities have a preference for residing in more integrated settings, but are unable to do so due to a lack of services to assist them to remain safely in the community and/or lack of opportunity to do so because of a diminished community support for community residential placements (Coalition, 2003).

At the policy level, social workers can also work toward an Olmstead plan that incorporates precautions against creating segregated communities filled with persons with disabilities. Gaining representation on the Olmstead planning task forces, either directly or through access to representatives on the task force, is one way to accomplish this. Social workers also have a role in disseminating related information to consumers and providers, as well as to community members and leaders who may fear having persons with disabilities living in their communities.

An integral role for social workers is to determine whether individuals they serve live in a segregated setting by choice or because they were denied options available to them under Olmstead, or perhaps were not aware these options were available. It is important that social workers referring individuals to more restrictive care settings know that they and their consumers do not have to settle for large community residences that may disrupt a community or crowd people of certain disability or age groups together. Even more importantly, social workers should be aware of the services available in the community and the service options made available through the Olmstead decision.

(3) Alleviating Fragmentation of Services

Continued fragmentation of public and private service provision systems will frustrate community integration efforts. In community mental health, for example, responsibility for assisting consumers to obtain clinical, medical, vocational, housing, educational, and·social support is often overseen by separate entities (Peele, 2000). Little coordination of services exists, unless one is fortunate enough to have case management. Similar fragmentation exists in services for seniors, people with developmental disabilities, children, and those with physical disabilities. People of all ages and with all types of disabilities cannot live in an integrated setting if only housing and personal care services are addressed. Social supports, spiritual supports, transportation, employment opportunities, and access to health insurance if disability begins to improve, are only a few of the supports and services that must be addressed.

An excellent model of a holistic approach to service delivery is New York State's well-established Willowbrook Class case management system. Willowbrook case managers are responsible for coordination of services for individuals with developmental disabilities who once lived at the Willowbrook Developmental Center, an institution that was the subject of a media exposé and subsequent congressional scrutiny during the 1970s for neglectful and abusive treatment of residents. With caseloads capped at twenty consumers, Willowbrook Class case managers are overseen by state-appointed paid Willowbrook advocates to assure that each former Willowbrook resident's best interests, including maximal opportunity to participate in the community, are consistently met (Finding Aid, 2005).

This case management model benefits consumers through lower-than-average client caseloads and periodic congressional scrutiny. Willowbrook advocates have more specialized training than do case managers and, through state-appointed status, have greater access to services their clientele may need. A group of Olmstead case managers charged with the specific responsibility to maximize community integration, armed with special training, limited caseloads and specialized oversight, may have greater success in effectively implementing the Olmstead decision.

(4) Transitioning into More Integrated Settings

A key concern for states is assisting individuals making the transition from places such as jails, adult homes, and nursing homes in re-entering the community. It is imperative to avoid the devastation evidenced in the large-scale, ill-prepared state psychiatric hospital closures of the 1960s through 1980s. Many people who relocated from long-term hospitalizations were unable to acquire the services and supports needed to thrive in the community. They ended up in different institutions less able to meet their needs, e.g., adult homes, or even on the streets where they may have spent years without proper services (Coalition, 2003; Herbert & Young, 1999; Peele, 2000).

The crisis for at least some people with mental illness living in adult homes where their service needs went unmet illustrates how harmful ill-planned community integration movements can be. People presently living in institutions need to develop or re-learn basic skills such as budgeting, self-determination of services, basic decision making, cooking, and housekeeping to support successful community placement (Velgouse, 2002). These persons also need to be linked with appropriate ongoing services in the community. For this to happen, professionals aiding in these transitions need to be sure that these services actually exist, and if not, assure that such services can be developed under Olmstead. The majority of states currently have no such programs to aid in an incremental and successful transition from institutional settings to community settings (Velgouse, 2002). Social work professionals are in a unique position to design and advocate for programs that would address these needs.

(5) Assuring Continuous Funding During Life-Stage Transitions

Implementing transitions across funding streams for people with disabilities during major developmental and level of care transitions has traditionally been a barrier to full and meaningful community integration. For example, toddlers moving into school years, children aging into adulthood, and adults transitioning into senior status are at risk of losing services due to changes in funding streams. No adequate system of orderly transition to different streams of funding exists. This is also true in aging services. Older people being served in the community under long-term care often also need medical care. Medicaid often covers long-term care, while Medicare generally pays acute health care. Coordination of benefits in the present system is extremely difficult and often leads to unnecessary reimbursement denials and lack of needed services to remain in the most integrated setting (Chevalier, 2002).

Social workers are often the ones who must piece together the services for these individuals. A few states, including Texas, are experimenting with a money follows the person system, in which funds are allocated to a person based on need or disability rather than the particular service delivery system with which the person is engaged (Crispell et al., 2003; NCSL, n.d.). Several related federal legislative initiatives have been and are currently being introduced, but to date, none have passed. However, The White House's New Freedom Initiative and Executive Order 13217 both strongly encourage this type of person-centered funding stream (HHS, 2003 a & b; White House, 2001); both could potentially be major advocacy tools for social workers nationwide.

(6) Creating Comprehensive Assessment Tools

Pursuant to the Olmstead mandate, comprehensive universally applicable assessments to determine the most appropriate and integrated setting for an individual must be developed (Cohen, 2001; LII, 1999). Olmstead is very far-reaching and applies to infants, children, young and middle-aged adults, and seniors with cognitive, mental, medical, and other physical disabilities.

Developmentally appropriate assessment tools for many different types of disabilities must be developed that are culturally sensitive and can be translated into the primary languages spoken across the country. Professionals must be trained to conduct assessments once validated and standardized.

Social workers are well trained in assessment and able to identify many types of needs, including basic needs for food, housing, and medical care, as well as need for companionship, spirituality, physical and emotional safety, self-esteem, and maximum interdependence. In many fields, a social worker will be one of the first professionals to see an individual and is in an excellent position to conduct these assessments (Mattaini & Kirk, 1991). Hence, social workers can be pivotal players in Olmstead implementation through designing comprehensive assessments of capability for community living, as well as level of consumer interest in long-term options.

(7) Addressing Workforce Shortages in Community-Based Services

Individuals and families find it exceedingly difficult to cope with rapid staff turnover and shortages. Workforce shortages for direct care workers must be overcome in order to provide needed services to individuals in their homes and communities. Direct care workers tend to be underpaid, under-insured, poorly educated, and lack educational and promotional opportunities (Coalition, 2003; Coleman, 2002; HHS, 2003a; HHS, 2003b). Suggestions to improve job retention and aid training include student loan deferments, educational grants and certification programs. State subsidized health insurance programs would improve accessibility of health insurance for under-insured direct care staff. Some states have innovatively allowed reimbursement of non-immediate family members who provide services in the home or allow consumers to hire their own staff with family support services reimbursement funding (Davis et al., 2002; HHS, 2003b; NAPAS, 2002; NCSL, n.d.). Social work professionals should examine local workforce issues and legislative initiatives that may impact the workforce shortage and retention issues. Olmstead-related initiatives should include a workforce feasibility evaluation with consideration for the funding of staffing initiatives. To neglect the staffing aspect of Olmstead initiatives may lead to people languishing underserved in their communities.

(8) Balancing Community-Based and Institutional Services

Attaining a balance between community-based and institutional services over time is a crucial component of any feasible Olmstead plan. Nationally, a strong institutional bias has existed since early colonial days (Perlin, 2000). Medicaid and Medicare each have a historical institutional bias, which created an imbalance in options available to persons in the community (HHS, 2003a). Availability of service providers is also biased toward institutions. Due to direct care workforce shortages, it is often difficult to find reliable home health care staffing to provide the services necessary to keep people out of institutions. Hence, people with disabilities often are forced into rehabilitation centers or nursing homes.

Eligibility criteria for community-based services, such as in-home nursing care, can be daunting. People must often be homebound to receive certain services, creating an isolating experience for people who desperately need services but are unable to leave their own homes, even with aid of family or other informal supports (Coalition, 2003; HHS, 2003; Johnson & Bowers, 2002). Likewise, in many states, including New York, home care agencies will refuse to provide services to persons with disabilities, stating they are inappropriate for or unsafe in their own homes (Coalition, 2003).

Present day institutional bias is reinforced by financial disincentives (Batavia, 2002; Coalition, 2003; Perlin, 2000). For example, in many states, counties must match funds for community-based services but not for institutional care, often leading to incentives to place people in institutions rather than maintain them safely in their communities. Additionally, projected increases in the total numbers of older adults and persons with disabilities living into older age will tax existing community-based services, which are already plagued by long waiting lists and short staffing. Closely connected is the issue of resistance to maximal community integration of persons with disabilities by corporate health care and other interests (NCSL, n.d.). Convincing political, corporate and other interests that Olmstead-related changes is in the best interest of those served by the programs will be a daunting task. To accomplish this goal, social workers must understand arguments against change being presented by these and other groups and be prepared to offer a response.

One route to reduce the institutional fiscal bias in states' long-term care programs recommended by the federal government is to tie funding to individual people rather than service agencies so that the money follows individuals into the community (HHS, 2003a; NCSL, n.d.). New York's task force, for example, recommends transitioning people living in adult homes into the community through re-allocation of state-shared funding from adult homes into housing subsidies specifically for those leaving adult homes for more integrated settings (Coalition, 2003). Olmstead task forces and advocacy groups in other states recommend slowing or altogether ceasing funding for new nursing home beds and instead using funds that would have been put into new nursing home beds into community services to support transitioning individuals. States would then transition people out of nursing homes who could be more appropriately served in the community, and individuals assessed to need institutional care could fill open beds (Coalition, 2003).

Social work professionals will need to evaluate the efficacy of these types of plans in order to effectively advocate for the best possible balance in a given state. It would not be practical to altogether cease funding to nursing homes. Addressing the mortgage/financial impact on nursing homes and the retraining and reallocation of staff are also important concerns. Social workers must understand that effectively influencing Olmstead policymaking involves delivering practical alternatives and empirical evidence as to why posited plans make sense to implement.

(9) Quality Assurance Activities

How to provide effective quality assurance in Olmstead activities when there is a desire to balance mandates with state flexibility presents pressing issues. Social workers can play a pivotal role in the quality assurance plans related to Olmstead activities by advocating for plans that reflect the needs of their constituencies. This will not be an easy task, since the population covered under Olmstead is very diverse. Annual audits of Olmstead-related implementation and evaluations should be conducted.

Social workers with intimate knowledge of the needs of people with disabilities in their states must be involved in these evaluations. Quality indicators used in evaluation should include consumer satisfaction surveys, wait lists, funding allocation, numbers of people in community settings, and available community and institutional services. In addition, audits of Olmstead case management charts, reviews of complaints and litigation, and reviews of where states stand in meeting their Olmstead objectives should be included. Annual reviews should be available to the public, much as state school report cards are through the Education Department. Social workers can use these reviews to influence not only the implementation of Olmstead, but also future amendments to policy. What is not accomplished in the influence of current Olmstead planning can still be pursued as policy is reviewed and revised through these mechanisms.

(10) Forging Cross-Disability Collaboration

Though the Olmstead decision was based upon a case of two institutionalized women with mental illness and developmental disability, it covers all individuals with all disabilities, of all ages (Johnson & Bowers, 2002). It is imperative that all eligible individuals have equitable access to Olmstead-based community resources. There is a risk that advocates will fight for their constituencies and lose opportunities to increase their influence and strength through cooperation with other disability groups. This holds true of groups representing the same disability interests, but perhaps having different beliefs on how to attain their goals. The social work profession is represented in all disability arenas and thus can aid in forming and supporting collaborative efforts. To do so will require that social workers join together in the common cause of Olmstead implementation.

(11) Funding State-Level Olmstead Initiatives

Without adequate funding, Olmstead related policy initiatives, no matter how well planned, stand little chance of making an impact on community integration. Recent budget deficits have created a disincentive for states to implement an effective Olmstead plan. With the current fiscal crisis, alternative choices for funding Olmstead-related activities must be proposed (Coalition, 2003; Kafka, 2002).

A number of federal funding sources exist to assist states in Olmstead implementation. Taken together, a package of grants can take states a long way toward implementing and funding a comprehensive Olmstead plan. For example, additional waivers may be created for people with mental illness, children with emotional disturbances, and people with degenerative conditions. Existing waivers might be expanded for older adults and people with developmental disabilities.

In addition, Real Choice System Change Grants can aid in design and implementation of community integration efforts. Nursing Facility Transition Access Grants can be used to aid in transitioning people out of nursing homes into the community and Community Integrated Personal Assistance Services and Support Grants increase the availability of personal assistance to individuals with disabilities living in the community (HHS, 2003a; HHS, 2003b). Grants are also available to specific administrative agencies, such as departments of justice, education, and labor to fund specific areas of community integration. These are only a few of the federal grant opportunities available to states, many of which are earmarked for performance of certain Olmstead-related goals. Alone, each of these grants may not always offer a significant amount of money state by state, but creative combinations can lead to a comprehensive funding package. Social workers must advocate for such creative and innovative approaches.

(12) Engaging in Public Advocacy

The response to the Olmstead decision must be comprehensive and sustained if real change in long-term care is to be realized. Contributing to such a sustained response through ongoing public advocacy is a critical social work role. Olmstead cannot remain a nebulous regulation or decision known only to attorneys, lobbyists, and politicians. It needs to become as well known by the media and the public as Social Security and welfare. Social workers are in a unique position through their history of community organizing to take the lead in this endeavor.

For this to happen, the importance and far-reaching impacts of Olmstead must be communicated in such a way as to capture people's interest. Other advocacy organizations such as state chapters of AARP, NAMI, Mental Health Association, ADAPT, The ARC of the United States, and organizations representing individuals with physical disabilities can be powerful partners in educating the public and other advocacy organizations. A social work-led educational initiative should elicit recommendations for Olmstead implementation, measure the feasibility of such recommendations and suggest ways in which the public can advocate for change.

Social workers should also work to dispel stereotypes of people with disabilities. For instance, developmental disabilities advocates have been successful in many instances in educating local communities that having community residences in a neighborhood is not dangerous and does not lower property values (Davis et al., 2002). For example, the Florida Developmental Disabilities Council partnered with the Florida Housing Coalition in a special needs housing demonstration project to develop strategies for successful community integration. Key strategies that were found to be most successful included education, purchase of existing single family homes rather than building new large homes, keeping number of residents under four, and efforts to keep support staff travels as non-intrusive as possible (LIHS, 2002). It will be important to learn about such successes and attempt to replicate them for other community projects that integrate people with all types of disabilities into the community.

Once a plan is created, social workers need to assure buy-in from politicians and other interest groups. HHS and CMS have promised states more flexibility in Medicaid and Medicare funding to implement Olmstead (HHS, 2003a; HHS, 2003b). However, states may be resistant to change, and social workers should work with states on identifying the benefits of Olmstead implementation. Advocates and consumers must also partner to educate corporate health care lobbyists and business groups on benefits of increased community-based services. For example, such interests stand to benefit from expanded community funding to create and manage new and existing services, as well as by infusion of new consumers into local communities. This can more than offset losses due to de-institutionalization.

CAUTIONS

The importance of an incremental approach to planning and implementation cannot be over-emphasized. Hard numbers should be used in the plan's target objectives. Goals for Olmstead implementation will need to be broken down into measurable incremental objectives with time frames. These should reflect the needs for legislation, for the identification of funding alternatives, and for the purposeful transition of both consumers and resources into community alternatives in a time frame that engages, rather than alienates, stakeholders.

Social workers must also be vigilant of unintended consequences as implementation proceeds. Unintended consequences may include, but are certainly not limited to, inadvertent community segregation into large group homes, isolation of people with disabilities in their communities, increased burdens on local provider agencies to provide community-based services with too few staff, resources, and low reimbursement rates (Bazelon, n.d.b.; Chevalier, 2002; Coalition, 2003; NAPAS, 2003). Efforts should be made to assure that states' Olmstead task forces remain in existence long enough to address these unanticipated consequences. Some groups may have been left out of the initial planning phases; advocates should strive to assure that this does not happen and that such groups are included in later stages so that no stakeholder is disenfranchised from Olmstead planning. The best way to keep people invested is through knowledge dissemination and by providing recommendations for action that social workers, providers, and consumers can take.

CONCLUSIONS

For social workers to effectively carry out these roles, they themselves must be informed about the Olmstead decision and its implications for clientele of all ages with all types of disabilities. Social workers must also be engaged in Olmstead planning and implementation processes. Social work organizations, continuing education programs, and degree programs need to provide tools to build the skills outlined here, such as public advocacy, quality assurance, and addressing barriers to persons with disabilities living in the most integrated setting in their communities. Individual social workers can be active on Olmstead-related task groups and advisory meetings. The opportunity afforded by the Olmstead decision to radically change long-term care delivery should not be missed.

NOTE

1. Post-Olmstead litigation is an important source of information for assessing how the legal system is interpreting and applying the Olmstead Decision. In the first year alone, over 200 complaints were filed. While detailed discussion of Olmstead litigation is outside the scope of this article, it is hoped that these brief illustrations will give the reader a sense of how the Olmstead Decision is being operationally defined by courts, states and persons with disabilities and their advocates. To learn more about Olmstead litigation, visit the Health and Human Services (HHS) Office for Civil Rights web site, www.hhs.gov/ocr/complianceactiv.html.

REFERENCES

Bartels, S. J., Miles, K. M., Dums, A. R., & Levine, K. J. (2003). Are nursing homes appropriate for older adults with severe mental illness? Conflicting consumer and clinician views and implications for the Olmstead Decision. *Journal of the American Geriatrics Society, 51*, 1571-1579.

Batavia, A. I. (2002). Consumer direction, consumer choice, and the future of long-term care. *Journal of Disability Policy Studies, 13*(2), 67-73.

Chevalier, L. (2002). *Promising practices in home and community based services*. Retrieved February 6, 2003, from US Centers for Medicare and Medicaid Services, The MEDSTAT Group, Web Site: *http://www.cms.gov/*.

Coalition for the Aging. (February 2003). *Developing a comprehensive effectively working Olmstead plan in New York State*. Retrieved February 28, 2003 from *www.coalitionforaging.org*.

Cohen, P. S. (2001). Being "reasonable": Defining and implementing a right to community-based care for older adults with mental disabilities under the Americans with Disabilities Act. *International Journal of Law and Psychiatry, 24*, 233-252.

Coleman, B. (2002). *State legislatures and Olmstead: What's new in 2002*. Retrieved March 24, 2003 from *http://www.ilru/org/online/handouts/2002/donlin/coleman.html*.

Crisp, S., Eiken, S., Gerst, K., & Justice, D. (2003). *Money follows the person and balancing long term care systems: State examples*. Retrieved March 23, 2003 from *http://www.os.dhhs.gov/*.

Davis, D., Fox-Grage, W., & Gehshan, S. (n.d.). *Deinstitutionalization of persons with developmental disabilities: A technical assistant report for legislators*. Retrieved September 13, 2003 from *http://www.ncsl.org*.

Donlin, J. M. (2003). Moving ahead with Olmstead. *State Legislatures, 29*(3), 28-32.

Herbert, P. B., & Young, K. A. (1999). The Americans with Disabilities Act and deinstitutionalization of the chronically mentally ill. *Journal of American Academic Psychiatry Law, 27*(4), 603-613.

Johnson, H. M., & Bowers, L. (2002). Civil rights and long-term care: Advocacy in the wake of Olmstead and L.C. ex rel. Zimring. *The Elder Law Journal, 10*(2), 453-461.

Judge David L. Bazelon Center for Mental Health Law (Bazelon). (n.d.a). *Background on Olmstead v. L.C.* Retrieved on February 6, 2003 from *http://www.bazelon.org/ issues/communitybased/olmstead/lcbkgrnd.html*.

Judge David L. Bazelon Center for Mental Health Law (Bazelon). (n.d.b). *What the community integration mandate means for people with mental illnesses: The Supreme Court ruling in Olmstead v. L.C.* Retrieved on February 6, 2003 from *http://www.bazelon.org/issues/communitybased/olmstead/lcruling.html.*

Kafka, G. (2002). *Community first! Getting/Keeping people out of nursing homes and other institutions.* Retrieved March 24, 2003 from *http://www.ilru.org/online/handouts/2002/kafka/olmstead.html.*

Legal Information Institute (LII). (1999). *Supreme Court of the United States Case No. 98-536. Tommy Olmstead, Commissioner, Georgia Department of Human Resources et al., v. L.C., brought by Jonathon Zimring, guardian ad litem et al.* Retrieved March 24, 2003 from *http://www.thomas.gov.*

Mathis, J. (2001). Community integration of individuals with disabilities: An update on Olmstead implementation. *Journal of Poverty Law and Policy, 11-12,* 395-410.

Mattaini, M. A., & Kirk, S. A. (1991). Assessing assessment in social work. *Social Work, 36(3),* 260-266.

National Association of Protection and Advocacy Systems (NAPAS). (October, 2002). *Three-year Olmstead v. L.C. progress report.* Retrieved February 19, 2003 from *www.napas.org/.*

National Association of Protection and Advocacy Systems (NAPAS). (2003). *Olmstead Plans: State strategies and plan oversight.* Retrieved February 19, 2003 from *www.napas.org/.*

National Conference of State Legislatures (NCSL). (n.d.). *The states' responses to the Olmstead decision: How are states complying?* Retrieved March 12, 2004 from *http://www.ncsl.org.*

National Low Income Housing Coalition (LIHS). (2002). *The Olmstead factor: Integrating housing for people with disabilities.* Retrieved September 15, 2005 from *www.nlihs.org/nimby/spring2002.pdf.*

Peele, R. (2000). Fragmented responsibility, deteriorating care. *Psychiatric Services, 51(5),* 557.

Perlin, M. L. (2000). "Their promises of paradise": Will Olmstead v. L.C. resuscitate the constitutional "least restrictive alternative" principle in mental health law? *Houston Law Review, 37(2),* 999-1054.

Rosenbaum, S., & Teitelbaum, J. (2004). *Olmstead at five: Assessing the impact.* Retrieved November 24, 2004 from *http://www.kff.org/medicaid/7105a.cfm.*

Smith, G. A. (2002). Status report: Litigation concerning Medicaid services for persons with developmental and other disabilities. Retrieved September 15, 2005 from *http://www.hsri.org.*

Smith, J., & Calandrillo, S. P. (2001). Forward to fundamental alteration: Addressing ADA Title II integration lawsuits after Olmstead v. L.C. *Harvard Journal of Law and Public Policy, 24(3),* 695-755.

The White House. (June 18, 2001). *Executive Order: Community-based alternatives for individuals with disabilities.* Retrieved February 6, 2003 from *http://www.whitehouse.gov/news/releases/.*

University at Albany, State University of New York, M.E. Grenander Department of Special Collections and Archives, Archives of Public Affairs and Policy. (2005).

Finding aid for the Willowbrook Review Panel records, 1968-1981. Retrieved September 14, 2005 from *http://www.albany.edu/speccoll/findaids/apap127.htm.*

U.S. Department of Health and Human Services (HHS). (2003). *Delivering on the promise: Self-evaluation to promote community living for people with disabilities.* Washington, DC: U.S Government Printing Office. Retrieved on February 28, 2003 from *www.gao.gov/.*

U.S. Department of Health and Human Services Press Office (HHS). (2003). *President will propose $1.75 billion program to help transition Americans with disabilities from institutions to community living.* Retrieved March 24, 2003 from *http://www.os.dhhs.gov/news/press/2003pres/20020123.html.*

Velgouse, L. (2002). *The Olmstead Decision: Responses and impact.* American Association of Homes and Services for the Aging. Retrieved March 29, 2003 from *http://www.aahsaA_org.*

doi:10.1300/J083v49n01_06

The Olmstead Decision
and the Journey Toward Integration:
The Evolution
of Social Work Responses

Fran Yong, MSW

SUMMARY. The Olmstead decision declared unnecessary institutionalization as discrimination and triggered an expansion of community-
based care for all people with disabilities including the elderly, thus
accelerating integration. Setting a context for Olmstead and related social work interventions, this paper describes the evolution of definitions
of disability and examines how social work has responded to the development of critical social policies aimed at increasing community integration. doi:10.1300/J083v49n01_07 *[Article copies available for a fee from
The Haworth Document Delivery Service: 1-800-HAWORTH. E-mail address:
<docdelivery@haworthpress.com> Website: <http://www.HaworthPress.com>
© 2007 by The Haworth Press, Inc. All rights reserved.]*

KEYWORDS. Olmstead decision, integration, health and long-term
care, persons with disabilities, older people, social policy, social work
interventions

[Haworth co-indexing entry note]: "The Olmstead Decision and the Journey Toward Integration: The
Evolution of Social Work Responses." Yong, Fran. Co-published simultaneously in *Journal of Gerontological
Social Work* (The Haworth Press, Inc.) Vol. 49, No. 1/2, 2007, pp. 115-126; and: *Housing for the Elderly: Policy
and Practice Issues* (ed: Philip McCallion) The Haworth Press, Inc., 2007, pp. 115-126. Single or multiple copies of this article are available for a fee from The Haworth Document Delivery Service [1-800-HAWORTH,
9:00 a.m. - 5:00 p.m. (EST). E-mail address: docdelivery@haworthpress.com].

Available online at http://jgsw.haworthpress.com
© 2007 by The Haworth Press, Inc. All rights reserved.
doi:10.1300/J083v49n01_07

INTRODUCTION

The 1999 Supreme Court decision Olmstead v. L.C. declared that medically unjustifiable institutionalization of persons with disabilities, who can appropriately receive treatment in the community and who have sought to do so, constitutes discrimination under Title II of the Americans with Disabilities Act (Title II of ADA). This decision prohibits state and local governments from discriminating against or excluding people from public programs by reason of their disabilities (119 S.Ct. 2176).

The Olmstead decision referred specifically to individuals with mental disabilities. However, it has generated considerable discussion about reorganizing the Long-Term Care (LTC) system for older people and people with disabilities (Allen, 2001; Desonia, 2003; Kapp, 1999; Rosenbaum, Teitelbaum, & Stewart, 2002; Velgouse & Dize, 2000). The decision has facilitated the efforts of the social work profession to establish integrated service delivery in places where clients live.

This paper attempts to identify patterns of integration as reflected in social policy and effected in social work interventions (as policy application), thereby suggesting future directions for social work practice. The focus of this paper is on disability policy, which underpins the Olmstead decision, and the view that people with disabilities, as a group, have not yet been integrated into the mainstream. As can be seen in Table 1, definitions of disability (from the Medical Model, the Independent Living Movement, Section 504 of the Rehabilitation Act of 1973, and Title II of the Americans with Disabilities Act and the Olmstead decision of 1999) in turn influence social work interventions–from casework, case management, and consumer direction to care coordination.

This paper takes the position that social/historical events have been primary influences on the evolution of policy/program initiatives and of related social

TABLE 1. A Framework on Evolution of the Definition of Disability and Social Work Intervention

Year	Ideology & Policy	Policy assumption	SW Perspective	SW Intervention
1950s	Medical Model	Individual inability	Pathology	Casework
1970s	Independent Living Movement	Social construction	Ecological	Case Management
1973	Section 504			
1990	Title II of the ADA	Functional limitation	Strengths	Consumer-Direction
1999	The Olmstead Decision	Social responsibility	Empowerment	Care Coordination

work interventions. There are therefore three key related questions in the post-Olmstead decision era: (1) Who has been integrated?; (2) How they will access the mainstream?; and (3) What barriers exist? These are addressed and suggestions are presented to reduce barriers to integration.

EVOLUTION OF DISABILITY DEFINITION: WHO HAS BEEN INTEGRATED?

Disability as an Individual Deficit: Pre-1960s

Prior to the 1960s, there existed a stereotype of persons with disabilities as nonproductive and a burden. This permitted society to confine and isolate persons with disabilities, particularly with mental disabilities, in remote institutions and other segregated facilities (Funk, 1987). Large numbers of men with disabilities, in particular after World Wars I and II, then encouraged policy makers and mental health professionals to focus anew on people with disabilities. Disability was increasingly defined as the inability of a person to perform certain activities of daily living (ADLs). The emergent disability policy of this era focused upon rehabilitative services and income supports, i.e., services to help persons with disabilities deal with their disabling conditions. Vocational Rehabilitation programs, immediately following WWI, were provided to all persons with physical disabilities, with the expectation that those who received services would return to the work force and be removed from public assistance programs. However, persons with mental impairments continued to be largely housed in public residential facilities such as asylums, hospitals, psychiatric hospitals, etc. (Berkowitz, 1987).

Disability as a Social Production– The Independent Living Movement: 1960s

Along with the civil rights revolution of the 1960s, The Independent Living Movement (ILM) offered similar promise of greater participation and integration for people with disabilities. The ILM philosophy assumes that environmental barriers and service delivery based on the Medical Model place the greatest constraints on people with disabilities and creates dependency. Ratzka (1994) suggests that the principles of ILM emphasize living in the community, regardless of age, type, or extent of disability and that people with disabilities should have the same range of choices as people without disabilities, in all aspects of their lives, to develop fully their potential.

Disabilities in the ILM view are the result of the interaction between individuals and their environment rather than as a result of individual deficiencies. The ILM focused on societal responses, discrimination and environmental constraints as the primary barriers preventing people with disabilities from living independently in their communities. The appropriate intervention, then, is to modify the environment to accommodate the needs of people with disabilities. People with disabilities are viewed as active and responsible citizens and interventions focus on addressing barriers.

The movement has been valuable in altering the widespread perception (under the earlier Medical Model) that people are disabled primarily by their physical and mental impairments (DeJong, 1979). It provides substantial guidelines for developing more empowering approaches to working with people with disabilities.

Disability as a Social Class: Section 504 of the Rehabilitation Act of 1973

Section 504 of the Rehabilitation Act of 1973 (Section 504) was the first federal legislation to prohibit unnecessary segregation of people with disabilities (Scotch, 2001). Section 504 prohibited recipients of federal funds from discriminating on the basis of physical or mental disability, utilizing the language of Title VI of the 1964 Civil Rights Act (Fleischer & Zames, 1998). Section 504 views people with disabilities as a social class (29 U.S.C. § 794), although there are major physical and mental variations in different disabilities, people with disabilities as a group face similar discrimination in society. The *class status* concept of Section 504 unified people with different disabilities. Any person with any impairment was a person with a disability and had a right to the same protection from exclusion and discrimination as any other. The class extended to inlcude people with developmental disabilities or mental illness, and people who are aging of concern, however, was that although Section 504 provides mechanisms for protection against discrimination, it protected the rights of people with disabilities only in cases where federal money was being spent and used the term handicapped which harkened back to an individual deficit model.

Disability as a Functional Problem: Title II of the ADA of 1990

Title II of the Americans with Disabilities Act (ADA) was a logical extension of Section 504 to be inclusive of all circumstances, including those in the private sector, and advances the protection of people with disabilities from discrimination as a civil rights issue and encourages a primary and more expansive responsibility of state and local governments for accessibility, design, administration, and other aspects of programming even when services are contracted to other parties.

The definition of disability in Title II of the ADA was the same as Section 504; however, the term handicapped in Section 504 was replaced with the term *disability*. Title II implied that society recognizes that stereotyping attitudes and environmental barriers are the main factors impacting disability, regardless of whether people actually have an impairment or are suspected of having one. Further, the definition of disability in Title II of the ADA focused on the degree of limitation caused by the impairment in one or more of the major life activities (e.g., eating, dressing, bathing) (42 U.S.C. § 12211). Society was therefore encouraged to focus on the consequences of disability instead of the causes. Jones (1991) suggests that the new definition was particularly important for older workers as it now became possible to include many chronic conditions more prevalent with age.

Along with the positive aspects of Title II of the ADA, there were negatives. Title II did require that reasonable modifications be made in public programs that served qualified persons with disabilities in order to afford them an opportunity to receive services in the most integrated setting possible. However, Title II stated that public agencies did not have to "fundamentally alter" their programs in order to achieve such integration, although agencies were challenged to demonstrate why a requested alteration amounted to a fundamental alteration (Rosenbaum et al., 2002). Nevertheless, Title II of the ADA did create a least restrictive environmental standard, the most integrated setting, challenging the make-up of current Long Term Care (LTC) systems (Velgouse & Dize, 2000).

Disability as a Social Responsibility: The Olmstead Decision of 1999

The Olmstead decision of 1999 involved two women in Georgia with mental retardation and mental illness. They were institutionalized in a Georgia state hospital, and desired to live and receive treatment in their communities when their situation had stabilized. The Georgia state treatment professionals agreed to their request for community placement. However, they remained institutionalized long after their request. The Supreme Court ruled that Georgia discriminated against the two women based on their disabilities, thus violating Title II of the ADA:

> No qualified individual with a disability shall, by reason of such disability, be excluded from participation in or be denied the benefits of the services, programs, or activities of public entity, or be subjected to discrimination by any such entity. (42 U.S.C. § 12132)

Thus, the Olmstead decision became the next step in the embodiment of the recognition in Title II of the ADA, that all people with disabilities have the right to services in integrated settings. The Olmstead decision further specified the requirement that states follow the least restrictive environmental standard. The federal government issued new guidelines for states to comply with Title II of the ADA and provided grants to expand the availability of community-based services.

EVOLUTION OF SOCIAL WORK INTERVENTIONS

Social work interventions have been operationalized to address each policy leap, thus giving people with disabilities (including those who are aging) greater access to the mainstream (see Table 2). The evolution of social work interventions in health and LTC should be viewed as an accumulation rather than replacement process (Figure 1).

Case Work: A More Pathological Perspective: The 1960s. Casework was the primary delivery mechanism in disability services until the 1960s and was responsive to Medical Model ideas that individual deficiencies could be transformed and alleviated through the casework process. Only a qualified medical professional could bestow the labels *disabled*, and *old* often held a pathological implication. Persons with disabilities followed a treatment plan laid out by experts in rehabilitation medicine. The label itself facilitated the segregation of people with disabilities from their communities, and often isolated one group from another. In addition, services offered did not give attention to the strengths of people with disabilities (Stromwall, 2002). Yet there was an inconsistency for social work around values to improve the social functioning of each client, and the casework approach was criticized for contributing to depersonalization and fragmentation in health care (Rosalie, 1982). To the extent that aging was seen only in terms of managing the loss of independence, the casework approach also had a potential to contribute to depersonalization for this group. With the rise of the Independent Living Movement, criticism of casework mounted, encouraging a greater focus within the social work profession on influencing the environment.

Case Management: An Ecological Perspective: The 1970s. Although case management evolved from casework, its principles rely more heavily on the strengths of clients rather than their pathologies to the extent it was a movement away from the medical/deficit model, case a management emphasizes the case manager and client relationship, and that interventions addressing disability or aging needs should be based upon client self-determination and optimum receipt of services within a system (Rapp & Wintersteen, 1989). The ecological

TABLE 2. Examination of How Social Policy Influences Social Work Intervention

Policy (assumption)	Main Theme		SW Intervention (perspective)
	Management	Transformation	
Medical Model (inability/ deficit)			Case Work (Pathological)
Independent Living Movement	Alleviate the impact of harmful environment	Managed services within a benefit package	Case Management (Ecological)
Section 504 (Social construction of disability)			
Title II of the ADA (Overcoming Functional Limitation)	Reasonable modification	Increased role in making the decision within a specified system: proximal integration	Consumer–Direction (Strengths)
The Olmstead Decision (Social Responsibility)	Community integration	Coordinate in order to access the systems: Integrating consumer, providers, & setting	Care Coordination (Empower)

FIGURE 1. Evolution of Social Work Interventions

Case Work

Client's strength considered?   NO   →   Institutionalization

                YES

                 ↓

Case Management

Using external services considered?   NO   →   Case Work

                YES

                 ↓

Consumer Direction

Decision-making shared with   NO   →   Provider-driven case
consumers?   management

                YES

                 ↓

Care Coordination

Systems change?   NO   →   Provider-driven consumer
                                                  direction

---

perspective at case management's base appeared rooted in Independent Living Movement ideas focused on dynamic interplays between the individual and his/her environment. The social work profession thus shifted its focus to client strengths and improved transactions within the environment/community (Cox, 1992). Social work interventions ranged from de-institutionalization efforts to active development of community-based services to avoid institutionalization.

However, case management still placed a stronger emphasis on professional roles interacting with multiple systems that affect clients (Moore, 1990). An array of studies (Goering, Wasylenki, Farkas, Lancee, & Ballantyne, 1988; Hurley, Freund, & Taylor, 1989; Oktay & Volland, 1990) focused on the effectiveness of case management in reducing the cost of care rather than necessarily client valued improvements. There were also criticisms that the focus of case management was to reduce overall service delivery costs by offering services within a defined benefits package rather than in meeting the client's own needs (Bedell et al., 1997; Birne-Stone, Cypres, & Winderbaum, 1997).

Consumer Direction: A Strengths Perspective: The 1980s. Consumer direction based practice appears to be more responsive to both ILM and the non-discrimination aspects of Section 504. It was viewed as a way to afford consumers more choices and an increased role in decision-making. Consumer-directed programs reflected a strengths-based approach and did not require the expertise and judgment of professionals. However, consumer-directed programs did not always address the issue of lack of choices (Batavia, 2002; Stone, 2000; Velgouse & Dize, 2000).

Consistent with Section 504 and ILM perspective, consumer direction premises that LTC is predominantly non-medical focused on primarily low-tech services and supports that allow individuals with disabilities and/or the aging to function as independently as possible. Under this premise, two controversies arise over consumer-direction in LTC. Long-Term Care itself inevitably requires including acute and chronic care. First, ignoring the medical aspects ignores health issues for people with disabilities, an essential component of LTC (Binstock, 1992; Hill, 1999; Rosalie, 1982). Emphasizing strengths, and therefore independence, does not mean living without any assistance, help, or services. Taken to an extreme, with an increasing older population, the separation of health and social care may create problems for caring for older people living in the community.

The second controversy is that consumer direction should be based on sound information about service options and made in an environment in which viable choices exist (Wagner, 1996). However, people with disabilities and their families who seek LTC services face a confusing array of public and private services and providers. Difficulty in navigating these networks without assistance often means that people cannot find quality services, may spend too much money on the wrong services, and/or end up in a nursing home when their needs might have been met with community services (AARP, 2001). In addition, Kapp (1999) points out that many long-term care consumers may not be capable of or equipped for genuine consumer direction. The very powerlessness of the consumers who were the subject of the Olmstead decision to effect desired changes in their care illustrates this.

Care Coordination: An Empowerment Approach: The 1990s. The emergence of care coordination appears to position social work practice to support the desired consequences of the Olmstead Decision. Care coordination attempts to respond to consumer-directed concerns and is designed to support access to mainstream environments. The term *coordinate* is substituted for management and reflects recognition that many of the health concerns of older adults and people with disabilities have both medical and social components. Both information gaps and psychological barriers often keep older individuals and people with disabilities from appropriately using needed community programs and services (Ben-Sire, 1987; Waxman, Carner, & Klein, 1984). Care coordination is focused on the whole person, helping individuals to navigate an array of complex services and may facilitate delivery of quality care (Lawrence, 1988). It provides information about systems and offers linkages among systems. The underlying assumption inherent in the care coordination model is that the cross-training of professionals can help to increase both knowledge and exchanges, thereby potentially increasing consumers' access to systems.

Farel and Rounds (1998) suggest that care coordination may be a cost-effective approach to avoiding institutional care and urge the social work profession to design interventions that provide sound information in a timely and appropriate manner that assists consumers to connect to services in a way that maximizes consumer choice. Success also requires the development of an appropriate operational infrastructure (Fisher & Raphael, 2003).

CONCLUSION

Social policy and social work interventions are inevitably connected implying that policy weaknesses themselves may function as barriers to effective social work interventions. Society is becoming increasingly aging, and people who live longer than ever before have a higher probability of disabilities. A large proportion of these aging persons will need related services for their disabilities; community-based rather than institutional services will be expected and social work interventions must correspond and reflect the evolving policy framework. Understanding both the evolution of the policy context and its relationship to emerging social work practice both informs practice today and prepares social workers to consider the necessary evolution of both social work orientation and future interventions. With regard to social work interventions, case management practices are still prevalent and to some extent, so too are casework perspectives. Yet the evolving policy environment at least demands consumer directed perspectives and will benefit from care coordination practices. As responses to the Olmstead Decision continue to reshape views of disability, aging and long term care, social workers will need to consider how their own practice should continue to evolve in response.

REFERENCES

A.A.R.P. (1990). *A profile of older Americans.* Washington, D.C.

Allen, K. G. (2001). *Long-term care: Implications of Supreme Court's Olmstead decision are still unfolding.* GAO: United States General Accounting Office.

Americans with Disabilities Act of 1990, 42 U.S.C. § 12132, Olmstead, 527 U.S. at 616 Section 504 of the Rehabilitation Act of 1973, 29 U.S.C. § 794, The Supreme Court decision on Olmstead vs. L.C. 199 S. Ct. 2176 (1999).

Batavia, A. I. (2002). Consumer direction, consumer choice, and the future of long-term care. *Journal of Disability Policy Studies, 13*(2), 67-74.

Bedell, J. R., Hunter, R. H., & Corrigan, P. W. (1997). Current approaches to assessment of persons with serious mental illness. *Personal Psychology: Research & Practice, 28*(3), 217-289.

Ben-Sira, Z. (1987). Social work in health care: Needs, challenges and implications for structuring practice. *Social Work in Health Care, 13,* 79-95.

Berkowitz, E. D. (1987). *Disabled policy: America's programs for the handicapped.* New York, NY: Cambridge University Press.

Binstock, R. H. (1992). Aging, disability and long-term care. *Generations, 16*(1), 83-89.

Birne-Stone, S., Cypres, A., & Winderbaum, S. (1997). Case management and review strategies. In Alerine, R. M. and Philips, D. G. (Eds). *The Impact of Managed Care on the Practice of Psychotherapy.* New York: Brunner/Mazel Publishers.

Cox, C. (1992). Expanding social work's role in home care: An ecological perspective. *Social Work, 37*(2), 179-185.

Dejong, G. (1979). Independent living: From social movement to analytic paradigm. *Archives of Physical Medicine Rehabilitation, 60,* 435-446.

Desonia, R. (2003). Is community care a civil right?: The unfolding sage of the Olmstead decision. *National Health Policy Forum background paper.*

Farel. A. M., & Rounds, K. A. (1998). Perceptions about the implementation of a statewide service coordination program for young children. *Families in Society, 79*(6), 606-614.

Fisher, H. M., & Raphael, T. G. (2003). Managed long-term care: Care integration through care coordination. *Journal of Aging and Health, 15*(1), 223-245.

Fleischer, D. Z., & Zames, F. (1998). *The Disability Rights Movement: From charity to confrontation.* Philadelphia: Temple University Press.

Funk, R. (1987). Disability rights: From caste to class in the context of civil rights. In A. Gartner, & T. Joe (Eds.). *Images of the disabled, disabling images* (pp. 7-30). New York: Praeger.

Goering, P. N., Wasylenki, D. A., Farkas, M., Lancee, W. J., & Ballantyne, R. (1988). What difference does case management make? *Hospital and Community Psychiatry, 39*(3), 272-276.

Hill, H. (1999). Traumatic brain injury: The view from the inside. *Brain Injury, 13*(11), 839-844.

Hurley, R. E., Freund, D. A., & Taylor, D. E. (1989). Emergency room use and primary care case management: Evidence from four Medicaid demonstration programs. *American Journal of Public Health, 79*(7), 843-846.

Jones, N. L. (1991). Essential requirement of the act: A short history and overview. *Milbank Quarterly. 69*(1/2), 25-54.

Kapp, M. B. (1999). From medical patients to health care consumers: Decision capacity and choices to purchase coverage and services. *Aging and Mental Health, 3*(4), 294-300.

Lawrence, W. J. (1988). A care coordination system: Relief for overwhelmed patients. *Continuing Care, 7*(10), 29-31.

Oktay, J. S., & Volland, P. J. (1990). Post-hospital support program for the frail elderly and their care givers: A quasi-experimental evaluation. *American Journal of Public Health, 80*(1), 39-46.

Ratzka, A. (1994). The user cooperative model in personal assistance: The example of STIL, the Stockholm Cooperative for Independent Living. In E. Duncan & S. Brown (Eds.), *PAS in Europe and America: Report of an International Symposium*. NY: Rehabilitation International.

Rosalie, K. A. (1982). Lessons for social work from the medical model: A viewpoint for practice. *Social Work, 27*(4), 315-322.

Rosenbaum, S., Teitelbaum, J., & Stewart, A. (2002). Barriers to access to health care: *Olmstead v. L. C.*: Implications for Medicaid and other publicly funded health services, *Journal of Law-Medicine, 12*, 93-138.

Scotch, R. K. (2001). *From good will to civil rights: Transforming federal disability policy*. Second Edition. Temple University Press: Philadelphia.

Stone, R. I. (2000). Consumer direction in long-term care. *Generations, 24*(3), 5-10.

Stromwall, L. K. (2002). Is social work's door open to people recovering from psychiatric disabilities? *Social Work, 47*(1), 75-84.

Velgouse, L. & Dize, V. (2000). A review of state initiatives in consumer-directed long-term care. *Generations, 24*(3), 28-34.

Wagner, D. L. (1996). Consumer-directed services: An option for the future. *Perspective on Aging, 25*(2), 30-31.

Waxman, H. M., Carner, E. A., & Klein, M. (1984). Underutilization of mental health professional by community elderly. *Gerontologist, 24*(1), 23-30.

doi:10.1300/J083v49n01_07

NATURALLY OCCURRING RETIREMENT COMMUNITIES

History, Accomplishments, Issues and Prospects of Supportive Service Programs in Naturally Occurring Retirement Communities in New York State: Lessons Learned

Catharine MacLaren, LCSW, CEAP
Gerald Landsberg, DSW
Harry Schwartz

SUMMARY. Naturally Occurring Retirement Communities (NORCs) provide unique settings for the delivery of a variety of supportive services to the elderly. New York State's experience with the development of supportive service programs within NORCs provides valuable information for community planners and practitioners in terms of factors that

[Haworth co-indexing entry note]: "History, Accomplishments, Issues and Prospects of Supportive Service Programs in Naturally Occurring Retirement Communities in New York State: Lessons Learned." MacLaren, Catharine, Gerald Landsberg, and Harry Schwartz. Co-published simultaneously in *Journal of Gerontological Social Work* (The Haworth Press, Inc.) Vol. 49, No. 1/2, 2007, pp. 127-144; and: *Housing for the Elderly: Policy and Practice Issues* (ed: Philip McCallion) The Haworth Press, Inc., 2007, pp. 127-144. Single or multiple copies of this article are available for a fee from The Haworth Document Delivery Service [1-800-HAWORTH, 9:00 a.m. - 5:00 p.m. (EST). E-mail address: docdelivery@haworthpress.com].

Available online at http://jgsw.haworthpress.com
© 2007 by The Haworth Press, Inc. All rights reserved.
doi:10.1300/J083v49n01_08

contribute to the evolution and shaping of supportive service programs and lessons learned from existing programs. doi:10.1300/J083v49n01_08 *[Article copies available for a fee from The Haworth Document Delivery Service: 1-800-HAWORTH. E-mail address: <docdelivery@haworthpress.com> Website: <http://www.HaworthPress.com>* © *2007 by The Haworth Press, Inc. All rights reserved.]*

KEYWORDS. NORC, Naturally Occurring Retirement Communities, supportive service programs, elderly housing

BACKGROUND

The elderly population in America is increasing significantly and will continue to do so for the foreseeable future. By the year 2020, over 20% of the nation's population, about 51.4 million people, will be 65 years of age or older (Tilson, 1990). To put this in perspective, while the size of the entire American population has increased three times since 1900, the group aged 65 and older has increased *eleven* times (Vierk & Hodges, 2003). Along with many other cities and rural areas across the country, New York City is experiencing a phenomenon by which large numbers of people are aging in place and concentrating in certain neighborhoods, buildings, or housing complexes. This cluster of older people is called a "naturally occurring retirement community" (NORC). In 1985, Michael Hunt, a researcher at the University of Wisconsin, first coined the term "naturally occurring retirement community" and since then a body of literature has emerged addressing issues related to this trend.

NORCs have been defined as age-integrated buildings, housing complexes, or neighborhoods with large numbers of people 60 years or older. For buildings and complexes, the share of elderly is often half or more of all residents (Flanagan, 1992; Gozonsky, 1991; Hunt & Gunter-Hunt, 1985). As these neighborhoods and buildings were not originally designed for the elderly population, they do not inherently have the health, social, and other supportive services that older residents need in order to remain in place as they age. Nevertheless, most people have a strong desire to stay in their present communities and "age in place" (Tilson, 1990). Sources of this preference seem to be a desire to remain among a known social group, familiar surroundings, and a strong wish to preserve privacy and autonomy (Halper, 1980). A 1992 survey conducted by AARP showed that 27% of the nation's elderly live in NORCs and this share is undoubtedly increasing (Bertrand, 1995). One of their unique features is that they evolve rather than being created deliberately (Callahan & Lanspery, 1997). This evolution can occur because older residents move to an area, existing residents age in place, or younger residents move away from the area

(Marshall & Hunt, 1999). NORCs in urban and rural areas show different patterns and reasons for development.

Understandably, to meet the needs of residents, coordinated supportive service programs have begun to emerge and develop in NORCs (NORC-SSPs). NORC-SSPs are partnerships that bring together housing entities, residents, health and social service providers, government agencies, and philanthropic organizations allowing for flexible and varied services to promote independent and healthful living for as long as possible (Vladeck, 2004). According to Callahan and Lanspery (1997), NORCs offer significant opportunities for economies of scale in delivering services. Proponents of NORC-SSPs claim that the inherent cost savings are and will continue to be significant. The United Jewish Appeal (UJA)–Federation of Jewish Philanthropies estimated that in 1997 their on-site supportive services program at Penn South Mutual Houses forestalled 460 hospital and 317 nursing home stays, saving over $10 million for residents and taxpayers (Bell, 1999). Aging in place strategies can create a flexible system of supportive services that meets each elderly person's margin of need, rather than rigidly over- or under-serving the population (Lawler, 2001).

Recently, because of the rapid increase in the number of elderly people who are aging in place, government entities have begun to allocate resources for supportive service programs in naturally occurring retirement communities (NORC-SSPs). The 1994 New York State NORC-SSP legislation provided one million dollars in annual matching grants to facilitate making essential services readily available to NORC residents living in New York State by mandating the access of organized and accessible services (Brown, 1998). The first state public-private NORC-SSP Initiative administered by the New York State Office of the Aging (NYSOFA) focused on 14 low- and moderate-income housing developments where at least 50% of the heads of household (or, for the largest complexes, at least 2,500 individuals) were 60 years of age or older (Vladeck, 2004). New York City's newer program, begun in 1999, also provides matching funds to organized supportive services in NORCs (City of New York Department for the Aging, 2002). Both programs aim to make services more widely available to an increasing number of NORCs.

In the fall of 1999, with generous funding from the Fan Fox and Leslie R. Samuels Foundation of New York City, the New York University School of Social Work undertook the NORC Research and Education Study. One of the study's main objectives was to review current supportive service programs of naturally occurring retirement communities in New York State towards the goal of understanding the NORC-SSP history, development, challenges, successes, concerns, and potential lessons for others seeking to develop similar models in their communities. What follows are highlights of the information collected.

EMERGENCE OF SUPPORTIVE SERVICE PROGRAMS IN NORCs

As best as can be ascertained, between 1986 and 2001, professionally staffed supportive service programs for elderly residents were established in 35 naturally occurring retirement communities. Twenty-eight of those programs were in New York City; two in upstate New York, and five in other states. Information on the location, total number of housing units in the NORC, and the year that the program was established is shown on Table 1.

New York State's NORC-SSP has four objectives that have shaped subsequent programs. The first is to provide a range of flexible and integrated community-based health, social, and allied services that meet the varied need of consumers. The second is to stress preventive care and services that will enable elderly people to remain at home with independence and to avoid unnecessary long-term institutional care. The third is to give consumers and their caregivers an active role in the major decisions affecting their care. The last objective is to use the distinctive features of the naturally occurring retirement communities, such as the number and density of older people, to facilitate care and improve the delivery of services (Sources–see Table 1).

PROFILE OF SUPPORTIVE SERVICE PROGRAMS IN NORCs IN NEW YORK STATE

The size of the NORCs, which shapes the scope of the program, varies enormously, from 139 apartments in Troy/Mechanicville, to 15,372 at Co-op City in the Bronx, the largest cooperative in the nation. Likewise, the number of buildings ranges from one in Troy to 82 at the moderate density Clearview Gardens in Queens. The height of the buildings, from two floors in Troy to 38 at Co-op City, influences the efficiency with which services can be provided.

Many of the NORCs are moderate-income cooperatives and a few are rental housing. Close to 90% of the dwelling units are in moderate-income cooperatives. The population of the NORCs shows a wide variation from those composed largely of a single ethnic/racial group (white in the case of a single group) to those with sizable representation by several groups.

Table 2 displays information on the clients and the performance of the 14 supportive service programs that received funds at the time of the study from the New York State Office for the Aging. The information was compiled by NYSOFA from annual reports submitted by each program for the six years 1995 through 2000. The information enables the earliest years (1995 or 1997) and 2000 to be compared. Between 1997 and 2000, the number of care management clients, who receive the most intensive and time-consuming services,

TABLE 1. Naturally Occurring Retirement Communities with Supportive Programs for Elderly Residents

NORC	Location	Year Established	Total No. of Housing Units in NORC
Amalgamated/Park Reservoir	Bronx, NY	1995	1,400
Amalgamated Warbasse	Brooklyn, NY	1993	2,585
Big Six Towers	Queens, NY	1997	983
Center City Philadelphia	Philadelphia, PA	1992	c. 1,400
Chicago Commons Housing Co-op	Chicago, IL	2001	c. 500
Clearview Gardens	Queens, NY	1997	1,788
Co-op City	Bronx, NY	1995	15,372
Co-op Village	Manhattan, NY	1992	4,411
Deepdale Gardens	Queens, NY	2000	1,396
Forest Hills Cooperative	Queens, NY	2000	429
Greenbelt NORC	Greenbelt, MD	2001	1,600
Isaacs / Holmes Towers	Manhattan, NY	1995	1,173
Knickerbocker Houses	Manhattan, NY	2001	1,600
Lincoln-Amsterdam	Manhattan, NY	2000	1,444
Lincoln House	Manhattan, NY	2000	420
Metropolitan Cleveland	Cleveland, OH	1997	c. 1,200
Moore/Davenport–Troy HA Taylor Apartments	Troy, NY Mechanicville, NY	1997	139
Morningside Gardens	Manhattan, NY	1986	982
Northridge/Brulene/Southridge	Queens, NY	2000	1,578
Parkchester	Bronx, NY	2000	12,200
Pelham Parkway	Bronx, NY	2000	1,350
Penn South	Manhattan, NY	1986	2,820
Phipps Plaza	Manhattan, NY	2000	1,610
Crossroads Plaza Apartments/ Keeler Park Apartments	Rochester, NY		
Queensview/N. Queensview	Queens, NY	1997	1,090
Ridgewood Gardens	Queens, NY	2000	372
Ravenswood	Queens, NY	2000	2,166
Rochdale Village	Queens, NY	2000	5,600
Sheepshead Bay	Brooklyn, NY	2000	2,204
Spring Creek	Brooklyn, NY	2000	5,881
Trump Village Section III	Brooklyn, NY	1992	1,672
Trump Village Section IV	Brooklyn, NY	2000	2,800
Vladeck Houses	Manhattan, NY	1992	1,770
West Side	Manhattan, NY	2000	566
White Crane–Housing Co-op	Chicago, IL	2001	c. 600

Sources: NORC Supportive Service Center, Inc.; NORC Supportive Service Programs in New York City, United Hospital Fund; New York State Office for the Aging NORC-SSP, Program Reports, 2000.

TABLE 2. Selected Characteristics of Clients of Supportive Service Programs Funded by the New York State Office for the Aging 1995 and 2000

	1995	2000
·Care Management Clients		
Total	2,977 (1997)	3,610
Percent Female[a]	71	74
Percent White[a]	81	82
Percent Black[a]	12	9
Percent Other[a]	7	9
Percent Age 75+[b]	82	81
Percent Age 85+[b]	40	35
Percent Without Caregivers[b]	30	35
Percent One Person Households[b]	75	78
Percent Two Person Households[b]	21	21
Percent Three or More ADLs Activities of Daily Living[b]	37	35
Percent Three or More IADLs Instrumental Activities of Daily Living[b]	53	67
Nursing Home Stays Forestalled[a]	317 (1997)	404
Hospital Stays Forestalled[a]	460 (1997)	653
Group Service Participants[a]		
Total	71,083 (1997)	88,078

[a] For the entire year.
[b] For a sample month in the year.
Source: New York State Office for the Aging, NORC-SSP. Compiled from annual reports submitted by each program.

grew by 21% from 2,977 to 3,610. During the same period the number of elderly residents attending group services, such as social and educational activities, and health screenings, rose by 24% from 71,083 to 88,078. These increases, averaging 5% to 6% a year, occurred while the public funds available to the programs remained fairly stable (see Table 2).

The service programs reach the oldest, frailest and most isolated residents of the naturally occurring retirement communities. In both years about eight out of ten care management clients were 75 years of age and over and a large share (40% in 1995 and 35% in 2000) were 85 years of age and over. Upwards of three-quarters lived alone and another one-fifth with one other person, invariably their spouse. One-third cannot call upon someone (either a family member, neighbor or a paid person) for care. In 2000, over one-third were limited in three or more activities of daily living (ADLs), such as eating, walking or dressing. Two-thirds were limited in three or more instrumental activities of daily living (IADLs), like preparing meals, shopping, and managing their finances. Almost three quarters of the care management clients were women. The share of white clients remained stable over the six years, as the share of blacks declined and the share of others (i.e., Asians) rose from 7% to 9%.

Supportive service programs help elderly residents remain in the community and avoid or delay institutional care. In 2000, the programs reported that they helped forestall 653 hospital stays and 404 nursing home placements. Assuming that these residents were care management clients, this means that 18% of them benefited from forestalled hospital stays and 11% from forestalled placement in a nursing home. At these levels the financial savings to the public are substantial.

KEY FACTORS SHAPING SERVICE PROGRAMS IN NATURALLY OCCURRING RETIREMENT COMMUNITIES IN NEW YORK STATE

The key factors that have shaped the supportive service programs are antecedents of the program, planning and design, outreach and marketing, staffing issues, program services and delivery, program governance, volunteer and intern activities, role of the lead agency, partnerships with other agencies, linkages with other resources, financing services, management of the NORC and dynamics of the NORC.

Organized programs of supportive services for elderly residents do not simply appear in naturally occurring retirement communities. In some cases they stem from volunteer efforts of "neighbors helping neighbors." At times senior citizen clubs and other voluntary organizations in the NORC recognize that their members and other older residents need regular assistance in order to remain in their apartments. A crisis, such as fires in apartments or obvious and disruptive individual behavior, may prompt concerned residents, and/or the housing board and management, to take action and to obtain help for residents who are at risk. The availability of funds, such as those through State and City programs, may also be an inducement for organized services. The actual decision to start a program is made by the board of directors of a housing cooperative or the owner/manager of rental housing, often with advice from a social service agency.

Once the decision has been made to provide supportive services through a professional staff, the next step is to plan and design the program at the NORC. Written surveys and focus groups eliciting information on the characteristics and needs of elderly residents of the NORC are utilized. A number of programs use regular surveys for planning purposes. The experience of the agencies already providing services to elderly residents of the NORC and their understanding of the additional or expanded services needed by residents is important. The perceptions of volunteers, board members (especially elderly members), and management of the NORC regarding the services that elderly residents need in order to remain in the NORC are also a consideration.

The planning process for the program involves decisions in several key areas in terms of services to be initially offered and the priorities for meeting the social and health needs of elderly residents of the NORC: the lead agency for the program (if it is not already active in the NORC) and major partners; the initial budget for the program and the sources of funds and/or in-kind contributions; where the program will be located and adequacy of the location in terms of size, access to seniors, comfort and privacy; how the program will be governed, including the role of the board in cooperatives and the owners/managers of rental housing; and the division of responsibility between the housing entity and the lead agency regarding budgets, staff, financing, fund-raising, and outreach.

Program directors agree that marketing and outreach–informing elderly residents about services and encouraging them to use them–is one of their most important and often undervalued activities. If it is to be effective, marketing and outreach must start early and continue throughout the program. It should respond to changes in the NORC's population, such as the aging of residents and the arrival of new groups of seniors. Marketing and outreach are especially challenging with a diverse population and requires sensitivity to cultural differences and creativity in using appropriate techniques.

Potential techniques include distributed calendars of activities, monthly or quarterly newsletters, and flyers, multi-lingual in some cases, that advertise group activities, such as trips, and brochures briefly describing services and how to contact the program office. Events such as health screenings and fairs run by the program are excellent occasions for informing seniors about services. Some larger programs organize meetings in the lobbies of buildings where older residents can learn about the program and meet the staff. Designated floor captains can be very effective in informing older residents about services. Tables in building lobbies or in the management office can be used to publicize the program. Closed circuit television carries program calendars and other information.

The management office can distribute material, such as calendars, or combine it with rent or other management notices. Housing managers can provide the program with a list of the apartments occupied by seniors for direct outreach. Personal visits by the program staff are very effective in informing older adults about services. A neighbor, friend, family member, or management employee may recommend that a staff member contact and visit a senior. For reasons of privacy and respect for personal autonomy, these visits should be handled with discretion. Visits by a nurse or home chore worker offer opportunities to involve seniors in other services. Favorable word-of-mouth is an irreplaceable form of outreach. The lead agency and staff can market the program through community agencies and organizations used by elderly residents of the NORC. They may also participate in inter-agency councils.

Since most organized supportive service programs for seniors have been active for less than a decade, there is not a large pool of experienced workers to draw on. Nevertheless, most program staff worked with older people previously in, for example, home-based services, nursing homes, and senior centers. It's important to find staff who are motivated and flexible, have case management or group work skills, and are sensitive to the circumstances of the elderly. Bilingualism can be important depending on the population. Staff members are encouraged to participate in special training and to extend their knowledge. However, most training takes place "on the job," as staff learn from their colleagues by working with them, attending staff meetings and training sessions, participating in case work conferences, and through contacts with other agencies. Cases can be complex, involving mental and physical health and multiple ailments, and caseloads may be high. Salaries at supportive service programs are limited, especially when responsibilities are considered, and prevailing pay scales do not permit significant increases. Faced with these conditions, supervisors are called upon to recognize and support staff efforts and agencies to offer opportunities for advancement and professional education.

Variety, flexibility, and responsiveness are the hallmarks of successful supportive service programs in naturally occurring retirement communities. Each program has a different array of services, shaped by the nature of the NORC, the needs of its elderly residents, available resources, and the approach of the lead agency. The best way to view supportive services is to distinguish between those for individuals and those geared to groups of seniors, as shown on Table 3. In the realm of individual services, programs provide health and social services, such as care coordination; nursing care; home care; information and advocacy on benefits and entitlements; and referrals to other agencies. The most common group services are recreation, social activities, classes, and health information. In general, more seniors use group than individual services. Transportation deserves attention because of its importance and great

TABLE 3. Principal Services Provided by Supportive Service Programs Funded by the New York State Office for the Aging

Individual Services	Group Services
Coordinate and monitor health and social services.	Recreation: games, social dancing, movies, etc.
Referrals to health and social services.	Health screening: blood pressure, vision, hearing, cancer.
Health care: home visits by physicians and/or nurses; health care at NORC or at other agency.	Group purchasing: groceries, etc.
Transportation to medical appointments, etc.	Health promotion and education: nutrition, immunizations, accident prevention, stress prevention, etc.
Escort assistance: shopping, library, etc.	Support groups: caregivers, bereavement, memory loss, Alzheimer's.
Housekeeping and chore assistance provided or coordinated.	Trips outside of NORC: museums, concerts, shows, cemetery visits, shopping, etc.
Respite care for caregivers.	Classes, lectures and discussions: current events, men's and women's groups, etc.
Home care provided or coordinated.	
Emergency response systems.	Holiday celebrations and events; religious, ethnic, national, etc.
Long-term care planning.	Cultural classes: art, drama, music, writing, language, literature, etc.
Mental health screening, counseling, referrals.	Education: ESL, citizenship, computer.
Social adult day care.	Exercise classes: dance, yoga, aerobics, etc.
Financial management; legal assistance.	
Crisis intervention: home care, nursing, etc.	Outreach to residents through calendars, newsletters, flyers, visits, etc.
Friendly visiting, telephone reassurance.	Congregate breakfasts and meals.
Information, advocacy and counseling: benefits and entitlements: health insurance, home care, health care, long-term care.	Arts and crafts: knitting, photography, etc.
Home delivered meals.	

Sources: New York State Office for the Aging NORC-SSP, Program Reports 2000; brochures from individuals SSPs.

variation. Some programs have vans that take clients to dispersed services in neighborhoods where public transportation is thin. On the other hand, in neighborhoods where services are concentrated and transit is plentiful, seniors are more likely to make their own travel arrangements. Exceptional as is the range of services, the supply is often insufficient. The prime gaps are in individual care, the most expensive and labor intensive type of service. Adequate home care is a particular problem, sometimes enmeshing seniors in financial and regulatory barriers.

Programs at naturally occurring retirement communities exhibit their flexibility and responsiveness by expanding, adding, and even dropping services. Being small, local, and visible, programs can change services in response to "market conditions." A wide range of holiday observances are geared to the religious, ethnic, and cultural affiliations of elderly residents. When group services, such as some support or therapy groups, do not gain an audience they are dropped or the theme is changed to attract more clients. .

The major distinction in program governance is between naturally occurring retirement communities in cooperatives and those in rental housing. In cooperatives, which are self-governing and have traditions of mutual concern, participation in program governance is usually stronger and more articulated than in rental housing. Rental NORCs do not generally have a separate governing board or advisory council for the program.

The existing supportive service programs in cooperative NORCs can be divided into those that are incorporated as non-profit entities and those that are not incorporated. The incorporated programs are self-governing through their boards and are eligible to receive public and private funds. Incorporated as well as unincorporated service programs have advisory and other committees representing consumer and resident interests. The two most important forces in governance are the commitment of the board of the housing cooperative to the program and the involvement of advisory committees.

A number of programs grow out of volunteer activity. Most volunteers are "younger older" residents, although others sometimes join in, such as teenagers who tutor seniors in how to use computers. In a few programs, high school students escort seniors to local services and pay friendly visits. In addition to governing the programs, volunteers provide an enormous range of services, from the highly professional to the more common. For example, in some settings retired social and health workers offer care to other elders. Other personal volunteer services are escorting seniors to medical appointments, friendly visiting, telephone reassurance, and entitlement counseling. Volunteers also run group activities, including exercise classes, discussion groups, cultural sessions, social events, and support groups.

Some programs use social work and nursing interns from local universities. Supervised by the professional staff, interns enable the program to reach more residents and to offer more hours of service. Social work students perform case management as well as counseling during their placement. Nursing students visit seniors at home, where they administer medication, monitor health, change dressings, and do other nursing services. At the program office they may see seniors who come in for blood pressure readings, other health checks, and for advice on health matters.

Lead agencies are responsible for the program at each naturally occurring retirement community, providing core services, leadership, and management. Core services include providing (or obtaining) and coordinating health, social services and home care, counseling, and information and group services. Management involves administering the program; staff recruitment, training and supervision; forming affiliations with partner agencies; reporting to the program's governing body; and raising funds. The lead agency may also furnish specialized services, although specialized services are often entrusted to outside agencies.

The relation between the lead agency and the program at the NORC can take one of several forms. The lead agency may be essentially identical with the program. In some cases the lead agency also operates other services at the NORC that are not part of the SSP. The lead agency may be a significant presence in the neighborhood and have experience serving seniors. Or it may be that a city-wide agency specializing in services for the elderly functions as the lead agency. Where the choice of the lead agency is not obvious, the board of the NORC may interview several candidates. A trusting and clear working relationship between the lead agency and the program's governing entity is important for a successful program.

Although programs regularly cooperate with other local agencies, partnerships, where the lead and other agencies fully collaborate, pool resources, and share information, are not too common. Partnerships mostly arise when the lead agency and the partner have a history of working together and share an interest in the NORC and its clientele. By far, the most common partnership is with a health care agency, often a hospital. Several lead agencies are partnered with the Visiting Nurse Service, which provides nursing care to elder residents and may also perform other health tasks. Hospitals and health care agencies offer the necessary and specialized services that are beyond the resources of on-site programs.

One of the resounding achievements of supportive service programs are the extensive and productive connections that they have formed with other agencies. These linkages are of two types: one is with individual agencies and the other is participation in inter-agency councils whose member agencies serve the wider neighborhood. These connections enable the programs to offer seniors a much wider range of regular and specialized services.

Financing is one of the most critical factors shaping supportive services in naturally occurring retirement communities. City and State funding are the largest single source of income for service programs in New York. Public funds must be matched by the NORC where the program is located and the lead agency. The level of the match varies for public and private housing under the City and State programs and some may be in-kind. Other sources of financing for the programs include funds from the NORC where the program is located, in accordance with City and State matching requirements (some NORCs raise more than their required share), philanthropic funds raised by the program's governing body (i.e., a non-profit corporation) or the lead agency, and membership fees paid by users of the services. Although individual services are free, some programs charge a modest annual membership fee, in the range of $10 to $20, for access to group services. Membership fees raise a modest amount of money and give seniors a sense of belonging to the program. There may also be user fees for group trips to shows, museums, and shopping malls. In some programs non-residents may attend group events, if space is available, for a fee. Funds may also come from residents of the naturally occurring retirement community through monthly "check-off" contributions that are added to cooperative maintenance charges (usually by seniors); contributions from families of seniors; annual fund raising events in the NORC; bequests from residents who benefited from the program (one form of bequest is an interest in a cooperative apartment); income from an endowment fund for the program; in-kind contributions by the NORC's housing management such as space for the program in an available apartment(s); copying and distributing flyers and notices and similar help; in-kind contributions by local agencies, such as space in senior centers for group activities; goods and services donated to the program by local merchants, or discounts to individual seniors; and earmarked public funds obtained through an elected official, such as a member of City Council.

The relationship between the service program and the management of the naturally occurring retirement community is an important and sensitive factor. It can range from mutually supportive to weak and even non-cooperative. It is most productive where management has been involved in establishing the program and plays a continuing role. Maintenance and security staff is in regular contact with older residents and can be instructed to alert management to seniors who may need help or to report hazardous conditions in apartments.

Population trends, advances in medicine, and changes in housing markets have formed the generation of older residents now living in naturally occurring retirement communities. Continuing changes in the occupancy of NORCs and their market context will affect the need for services and how programs are perceived by residents. As in the past, these changes are more likely to be felt in the self-governing cooperatives than in public housing, which is government-owned and not subject to the pressures of the housing market.

Cooperative NORCs are going through a number of changes that will influence the need for and provision of supportive services for their elderly residents.

For one thing, as older residents leave they are being replaced by younger families. Cooperative NORCs report that new residents are more diverse–ethnically, racially, economically, and culturally–than the households they are replacing. New, younger families may have their own ideas on how (and even if) the cooperative should spend its money on social services. If newcomers stay and age, their needs for supportive services may be different than the current generation of elderly residents. As the population composition of NORCs changes, public and private supporters may review their financial commitments to services for the elderly.

In recent years, a number of regulated cooperative NORCs have become or moved closer to market rate housing. This shift has elevated the turnover and price of apartments. Even in cooperatives where turnover and price increases have not been as steep, newcomers are younger, more affluent, and more diverse than the residents they are replacing. The younger, more diverse cooperators may be more interested in maintaining their value and the economic level of the cooperative than caring for older neighbors. Their interest may be more in services for children, such as child care and playgrounds. As several programs are discovering, inter-generational activities, like computer classes, are one way to bridge this gap and to bring different groups of cooperators together (Personal communication with staff and residents of NORC-SSP).

THE VALUE OF SUPPORTIVE SERVICES PROGRAMS IN NATURALLY OCCURRING RETIREMENT COMMUNITIES

Existing programs of supportive services in naturally occurring retirement communities under common management can teach us much about how community-based services for the elderly can be organized in similar settings to optimize effectiveness and usefulness to clients.

Physical Attributes of Naturally Occurring Retirement Communities

By virtue of its size and compact layout, a NORC is an ideal setting for delivering supportive services to the elderly. For the lead agency and other providers, the size and form of the NORC yields economies of scale in service delivery. For example, a home care worker can easily visit two elderly residents for four hours a day each, or four for two hours each day. In an emergency older people can be quickly reached. The form of a NORC also makes it easier for elderly clients to get to the program office and senior centers in the NORC. In most NORCs walking distances are reasonable (and street crossings limited), except perhaps in extreme weather. Most seniors can get to the program office and group service locations on foot. Ease of access and convenience makes it more likely that seniors will actually use services.

The Nature of the Service Programs

One of the most impressive achievements of service programs in naturally occurring retirement communities is their diversity, responsiveness, and flexibility. Each program is distinctive in responding to the elderly residents of the NORC and their circumstances. They are located where their clients live and are visible. Program staff listen to their clients and to the governing board as well as to the managers of the housing. Although mistakes will be made, the programs are generally small and resilient enough so that they can be absorbed and adjustments made. Modest size also means that the staff collaborates on cases and shares information. The distance between the director and staff is not great and the director participates in the work and knows individual clients.

Relationship Between Program Staff and Clients

A number of features contribute to generally healthy relations between program staff and clients. For one, the staff is located in the housing community and the program office is visible and accessible. Clients drop-in to talk to the staff and to get information on activities. Since many users of services live alone and may not have family or friends nearby, they can become dependent on individual staff members. The program may be their "frontline" connection to the outside world. Close ties between clients and staff has advantages as well as drawbacks. The staff member may leave or the client may demand more attention than the staff can reasonably offer, so incoming staff must be sensitive to this adjustment and make it as smooth as possible.

Social Contacts and Support Among Residents

It is generally accepted that active and varied social contacts contribute to healthy aging. Supportive service programs foster such contacts and engagement. Group services not only inform, educate, and offer channels for cultural expression, but they bring people together in a congenial setting and promote neighborliness and friendship. Program directors report that the social interchange of group activities is valued by many seniors. Service programs provide ample opportunities through group events, volunteer work, and informal encounters for older residents to meet and to form social bonds and friendships. The naturally occurring retirement community itself promotes casual meetings and contacts in buildings and on the grounds, on benches, and along walkways. Neighborliness and mutual help among residents may also be encouraged by organized activities.

Role of Residents in Program Decisions

Service programs in naturally occurring retirement communities offer residents (and users) an active role in decisions affecting the program. In addition to the participation mandated by the agencies administering the programs, there are two other reasons for the involvement of residents in program decisions. The general reason is that the programs are located in defined housing developments and serve a limited and identifiable clientele. With their on-site location and visibility, they recognize that they are more accountable to their clients than other community-based services and must accord elderly residents a voice in program decisions. The origin of many programs in cooperatives, through volunteer efforts or action by the board, plus the fact that they are paying part of the cost, assures that residents are involved in decisions affecting the program.

Although it is not nearly as strong as in cooperatives, elderly residents of NORCs in rental housing have a voice in decisions affecting the program. In rental housing the interests of elderly residents tend to be represented through the tenant council for the entire development, rather than by an organization dedicated to the program. Even with this diluted involvement, elderly residents are more actively represented in this program than in other community-based services for older people.

Housing Management Serves the Interests of Residents and the Program

One of the most valuable and distinctive aspects of the service programs is the role of housing management in supporting the program and advancing the welfare of elderly residents. Although cooperation between management and the program varies, from constant to intermittent and weak, some degree of cooperation is always present. Management can advance the program in many ways: for instance by facilitating outreach, providing space, and identifying residents who may need services. Reciprocally, the program assists management by resolving problems that it has difficulty handling, such as disruptive behavior, dangerous conditions, or financial arrears that may undermine the operation of the NORC.

Collaboration with Other Community Resources

Service programs in NORCs depend heavily on other agencies to meet the diverse and shifting needs of their clients for individual assistance. Without outside resources many of their clients would not have the specialized services, such as adult day care and mental health counseling that they need to remain in the NORC. After establishing connections with outside agencies, programs refer clients and follow-up the results. Knowledge of and reliable contacts with outside agencies are important for successful referrals and care. Collaborations with outside agencies evolve and may change if expectations are not fulfilled.

CONCLUSION

As Americans age, new paradigms are emerging around how best to accommodate and care for the elderly during their "second phase of life" (Weiss, 1995). It is clear that many unique and specialized issues arise in providing supportive services in a NORC setting. The dearth of currently available literature is evidence of the tremendous amount that remains to be done to facilitate community-based services for clusters of elderly people. It is hoped that resources will continue to be allocated towards discovering effective and efficient means for providing services to those who need them to promote healthy, aging in place living. There is still a great deal more to learn about serving older people effectively in the community but NORC-SSPs appear to be viable, cost-effective models of service delivery.

REFERENCES

Bell, A. (1999, December). Aging placefully. *City Limits,* 5.
Bertrand, D. (1995, March 19). Program cares for co-op's seniors. *The Daily News.*
Brown, K. S. (1998). Elder care legislation. *The Gerontologist, 37,* 511-517.
Callahan, J. J., & Lanspery, S. (1997). Can we tap the power of NORCs? *Perspective on Aging, 26,* 13-20.
City of New York, Department for the Aging. (2002). *General standards for NORC supportive service programs.* New York: Author.
Flanagan, B. (1992). New options for retirement living. *New Choices for Retirement Living, 32,* 28-31.
Gozonsky, M. (1991). Look at naturally occurring retirement communities (NORCs). *Perspectives on Aging, 20,* 33-34.
Halper, T. (1980). The double-edged sword: Paternalism as a policy in the problems of aging. *Milbank Memorial Fund Quarterly-Health Society, 58*(3).
Hunt, M., & Gunter-Hunt, G. (1985). Naturally occurring retirement communities. *Journal of Housing for the Elderly, 3,* 3-21.
Lawler, K. (2001). *Aging in place: Coordinating housing and health care provision for America's growing elderly population.* Cambridge, MA: Joint Center for Housing Studies of Harvard University.

Marshall, L. J., & Hunt, M. E. (1999). Rural naturally occurring retirement communities: A community assessment procedure. *Journal of Housing for the Elderly, 13,*19-34.

Tilson, D. (Ed.). (1990). *Aging in place.* Glenview, IL: Scott Forseman & Co.

U.S. Census Bureau. (2003, October 16). *People: Aging.* Retrieved from *http://factfinder. census.gov.*

Vierck, E., & Hodges, K. (2003). *Aging: Demographics, health, and health services.* Westport, CT: Greenwood Press.

Vladeck, Fredda. (2004). *A good place to grow old: New York's model for NORC Supportive Service Programs.* New York: United Hospital Fund.

Weiss, J. (1995). Universities for the second phase of life. *Journal of Gerontological Social Work, 23,* 3-24.

doi:10.1300/J083v49n01_08

Integrating Services for Older Adults in Housing Settings

Carol S. Cohen, DSW
Elizabeth Mulroy, PhD, MSW
Tanya Tull, DSS
Colleen C. Bloom, RHP
Fred Karnas, PhD

SUMMARY. This paper draws on the work of the Housing *Plus* Services committee of the National Low Income Housing Coalition (to which the authors belong), constituted in 2000. The Committee is comprised of a diverse group of practitioners, administrators, policy analysts, professors, and researchers who share a commitment to the integration of services in housing settings. Committee members present their work, including the typology and principles discussed in this paper, at national conferences (NLIHC, 2005) and contribute to publications on the web (Housing *Plus* Services Committee, 2005a) and in print (Cohen, Mulroy, Tull, White, & Crowley, 2004), in order to disseminate the work of the NLIHC in this area and engage in dialogue with service providers, housing developers, and policy makers. doi:10.1300/J083v49n01_09 *[Article copies available for a fee from The Haworth Document Delivery Service: 1-800-HAWORTH. E-mail address:*

The authors acknowledge the work of the Housing *Plus* Services Committee of the National Low Income Housing Coalition, an organization dedicated solely to ending America's affordable housing crisis.

[Haworth co-indexing entry note]: "Integrating Services for Older Adults in Housing Settings." Cohen, Carol S. et al. Co-published simultaneously in *Journal of Gerontological Social Work* (The Haworth Press, Inc.) Vol. 49, No. 1/2, 2007, pp. 145-164; and: *Housing for the Elderly: Policy and Practice Issues* (ed: Philip McCallion) The Haworth Press, Inc., 2007, pp. 145-164. Single or multiple copies of this article are available for a fee from The Haworth Document Delivery Service [1-800-HAWORTH, 9:00 a.m. - 5:00 p.m. (EST). E-mail address: docdelivery@haworthpress.com].

Available online at http://jgsw.haworthpress.com
© 2007 by The Haworth Press, Inc. All rights reserved.
doi:10.1300/J083v49n01_09

<docdelivery@haworthpress.com> Website: <http://www.HaworthPress.com>
© 2007 by The Haworth Press, Inc. All rights reserved.]

KEYWORDS. Housing, older adults, assisted living, NORC, housing plus services, typology, principles

INTRODUCTION

Consider the following experiences:

- Charlene and Alfred Charles live in a privately owned apartment building in the area. Mrs. Charles is 78 years old, has a thyroid condition, and appears to have suffered small strokes. When she was referred to us, she had not seen her doctor in over 18 months and not taken any of her medications. This affected her mental health, as she was agitated and often did not make sense. Her husband is 87 years old with obvious signs of dementia. Their clothes were dirty and they appeared not to have bathed. Mr. Charles is a retired civil servant.
- Esther Rothman is a retired professional woman in her mid 80's. She has multiple medical problems which impact her mobility. When she was healthier and when her friends were driving, she was busy attending local concerts, lectures, and community events. However, this has become increasingly difficult. She is a member of our program's advisory board and brought up her concerns about getting around at a meeting.
- Rafael Brown, at 93 years of age, lives in an AR Residential Community. Next door to him lives Angela Murphy, who is 84. Mr. Brown was and is in notably good health, though he does not cook and never liked to eat alone. Mrs. Murphy has long been confined to a wheelchair and, though she loves to cook, was not always able to prepare meals. Both have been active supporters of the resident association and have been volunteering at the resident-run Country Store, located on the first floor of the building to provide convenient access to basic food supplies and additional niceties.

These vignettes share two important elements–each is a story about the experience of older adults and each relates to housing. However, the stories differ from each other in relation to the particular challenges these older residents encounter and the type of housing and service settings in which they reside.

This paper will build on these similarities and differences by first examining the literature linking older adults, housing settings, and services; next, describing the diverse community settings in which elders reside; and, finally, identifying and illustrating how common principles can guide effective delivery of services to older adults across settings and communities.

This paper draws on the work of the Housing *Plus* Services committee of the National Low Income Housing Coalition (to which the authors belong), constituted in 2000. The Committee is comprised of a diverse group of practitioners, administrators, policy analysts, professors, and researchers who share a commitment to the integration of services in housing settings. Committee members present their work, including the typology and principles discussed in this paper, at national conferences (NLIHC, 2005) and contribute to publications on the web (Housing *Plus* Services Committee, 2005a) and in print (Cohen, Mulroy, Tull, White, & Crowley, 2004), in order to disseminate the work of the NLIHC in this area and engage in dialogue with service providers, housing developers, and policy makers.

REVIEW OF LITERATURE

Linking Housing and Services for Older Adults

Housing is a key part of the social and physical environments of older persons because it represents physical safety, independent living, and access to social relationships and neighborhood resources (Pynoos & Regnier, 1991; Yeates, 1979). Housing becomes a critical environmental factor and social policy issue for society as people age and experience physical and mental decline. Current research shows that four out of five adults, now aged 65 and older are estimated to have one or more chronic health condition, such as hypertension, heart disease, or arthritis that may make living independently challenging. The potential effects of these illnesses on perceived quality of life and functional independence are alarming (Beattie, Whitelaw, Mettler, & Turner, 2003). In addition, due to cost and/or insurance issues, more often doctors and hospitals are releasing clients "quicker and sicker" (Grimmer et al., 2000, p. 1005; Linzer, 2002). This quicker release means that the elderly and their caregivers–if they have caregivers–are responsible for resolving their own health care problems at home, usually alone.

Research suggests that regardless of age, where one lives and with whom has a great impact on the economic, physical, and psychosocial well being of an individual (Mutchler & Burr, 2003) and has an impact on an individual's perceived quality of life. Historically, families took care of their own elderly members, or they were placed in residential treatment facilities. Multi-generational families have for centuries lived together and taken care of one another. But for many seniors in today's society, this is no longer the case. In today's fast-paced global environment, we have a generation of seniors who have always lived independently and often live very far away from their family members.

Today seniors do not necessarily want to move in with someone else or be institutionalized. If given a choice, most seniors want to stay in their own homes and *age in place*. Aging-in-place services refer to the concept of helping seniors resolve whatever problems, be they housing, healthcare, home care, home repairs, nutritional services, etc., that might affect that individual's ability to maintain his or her current living arrangement for as long as possible (Governor's Conference on Aging, 2004).

Aging-in-place is not a new concept; human beings naturally desire a place to belong and to have some value in society. Seniors are no different. Most elderly people do not want to see themselves as a *burden* to anyone, but as independent contributing members of society. At no time in human history is this more relevant than today. As the so-called *Baby Boomers* are reaching retirement age, many still potentially have 20 to 30 years of their lives left to live.

With much of the current gerontology research focused on caregiver issues and models of medical intervention (Stewart, 2003), service providers *do* have access to a wealth of information, if not a wealth of service options. Much of the current research indicates that many of the chronic diseases seniors deal with on a daily basis can be modulated by adapting healthy behaviors, reducing personal risk, and utilizing preventive clinical services including geriatric assessment and intensive care management (Beattie et al., 2003; Logan & Applebaum, 1995; Pynoos & Nishita, 2003; Struyk, R., Page, D. B., Newman, S. Carroll, M., Ueno, M., Cohen, B., & Wright, P., 1989; Van der Bij, Laurant, & Wensing, 2002).

There is long standing as well as rising interest and scholarly research in *appropriate* residential options for older persons as they become more frail. There is also concern over the lack of coordinated public policies that could facilitate the linkage of housing *and* services to help us prepare for anticipated growth of the aging population. Given these realities, there is a need for dialogue and action concerning the optimum quality of life we, as a society and a social work profession, want to offer the diverse elder population, and the frail elderly in particular (Beattie et al., 2003; Blieszner, 1986; Golant, 2003; Pynoos & Liebig, 1995; Toseland, McCallion, Gerber, Dawson, Gieryic, & Guilamo-Ramos, 1999).

HOUSING POLICIES
AND COMMUNITY-BASED SERVICE MODELS

Knowledge and technology generated by scholars and practitioners have offered a range of housing policy prescriptions for diverse groups of older persons and for effective models of *community-based services* that emphasize aging-in-place (Caplan, Williams, Daly & Abraham, 2004; Dear & Wolch, 1979; Ivry, 1995; Kornblatt, Cheng, & Chan, 2002; Pynoos & Liebig, 1995; Pynoos & Regnier, 1991). Pynoos and Liebig (1995) suggest that seniors need a wide range of residential options between (a) remaining in their own homes and residential care, and (b) connecting non-institutional alternatives with appropriate levels of care. Their central point is that housing and long-term care policies can no longer be treated as separate domains; housing is more than shelter, particularly for special needs populations, and long-term care must include housing as a key component.

The planful integration of housing for the elderly with its external community is one overarching element in Pynoos and Liebig's (1995) approach. They argue that seniors need to continue to live in–and be part of–their community and that a comprehensive linkage between housing and services would facilitate such aging-in-place. The aging-in-place process refers to seniors who receive needed services in the same place as their needs change (Mollica, 2003). These include seniors who live independently in their own homes, in senior housing, and in their communities with supportive services provided by outside agencies. The current continuum of care therefore needs to be changed, or at least broken down, so that elders would not have to move if they could get the appropriate in-home services. The housing emphasis is on personal residential *choice*, including: *staying put* (with modifications and services), house sharing, granny flats, foster care, and small group homes. Supportive housing can be substituted for nursing homes and, by restricting the building of nursing homes or converting existing nursing homes into residential settings that promote more privacy and autonomy, seniors could in fact have a housing choice (Pynoos & Liebig, 1995, pp. 8-13).

Policy makers with regards to community-based service utilization have supported this concept of choice. The Olmstead decision by the Supreme Court in July 1999 found that persons with disabilities, including the elderly, could not be limited to receiving care in an institution if community-based services were appropriate to their needs (Olmstead decision 28 CFR 35. 130[d] as cited in Mollica, 2003, p. 168).

This decision upheld the provisions of the Americans with Disabilities Act that requires states to provide the most integrated setting appropriate to the needs of qualified individuals with disabilities (Americans with Disability Act of 1990, P.L. 101-336, 104 Stat. 327).

However, while federal law says that, when appropriate, seniors have a right to community-based services, there are often not enough Community Based Organizations (CBOs) in the local community to meet demand. While individual states are not required to fully fund CBOs to meet local demands, they have an option to balance those needs with other financial obligations. Such balancing can lead to long waiting lists and a growing population of underserved elderly (Mollica, 2003, p. 166).

Such community-based models raise the question of *community capacity*–the presence of viable community-based organizations with the capability and partnership affiliations to adequately respond to an area's emerging and changing needs (Mulroy, 2003). According to Beattie et al. (2003), there are currently about 27,000 CBOs serving over 7 million seniors. However, information is scarce on CBOs and quality of life relative to elder population variables. The current research appears to be more universalistic and global in nature and supports the general hypothesis that as people age, they are likely to need in-home supportive services to maintain perceived quality of life and resist residential placement (Beattie et al., 2003; Caplan et al., 2004; Challis, Darton, Hughes, Stewart, & Weiner, 2001; Grimmer, Moss, & Gill, 2000; Golant, 2003; Kornblatt et al., 2002; Linzer, 2002; Logan & Applebaum, 1995; Mollica, 2003; Mutchler & Burr, 2003; Runciman, Currie, Nicol, Green, & McKay, 1996).

In sum, these themes in the literature suggest that a conceptual framework is needed to help practitioners and policymakers better understand and respond to the issues. The following Typology of Housing *Plus* Services is offered to help fill this gap.

TYPOLOGY OF HOUSING PLUS SERVICES SETTINGS

Terminology utilized in the field of housing development and operations is often confusing, even to people who work on housing issues on a daily basis. For those dealing with housing from a social services perspective, the complex language is even more problematic. It is therefore vital that there exists a means of communication on housing issues between the various sectors involved, particularly for those who are concerned with the delivery of needed services to an aging population in the community at-large (Figure 1).

To help simplify and demystify a complex set of often-overlapping terms in use across the country to describe a variety of housing programs linked to services, the Housing *Plus* Services Committee of the National Low-Income Housing Coalition has developed a *housing plus services* typology and matrix

FIGURE 1. Typology of Housing Settings of Older Adults (Housing Plus Services, 2005b)

Service-Enriched Housing: The term service-enriched housing has emerged over the past decade to define what is essentially a simple, adaptable mechanism to provide housing linked to services for the low-income population-at-large, living in private and/or non-profit housing settings including single family homes, cooperatives, and apartments. The major goals in service-enriched housing are to promote quality of life and improved social and economic well-being of residents, while encouraging community development, interaction, and interdependence. Residents of service-enriched housing may include any or all of the following: families with children, single individuals, disabled persons, extended families, couples, older adults, and people with special needs. While not necessarily targeted to older residents, the fact that crisis intervention and services coordination are available make this a viable housing option. Service-enriched housing can expand limited housing options for older residents, including the frail elderly, by providing a simple, cost-effective means for the delivery of supportive services in the community at-large. This model also supports *aging in place.*

Public Housing: Public Housing refers to housing publicly funded and owned through the Federal Department of Housing and Urban Development (HUD). However, public housing also refers to housing that is privately owned by either nonprofit or for profit entities and made affordable through Section 8 vouchers or certificates. The major goal of public housing is to provide affordable housing for low-income populations, including families with children, individuals, disabled persons, people with special needs, extended families, couples, older adults, etc.

Naturally Occurring Retirement Community (NORC): A national initiative, a NORC is identified as a community with a significant number of households headed by adults 60 years of age or older. Most recently, this term has evolved, to describe *aging in place*, with services most often provided by an outside senior services agency or program. These programs serve senior residents of intergenerational communities where seniors live in large numbers. The concept centers on developing supportive services programs for these seniors to access so that they can remain living in their neighborhoods. States have enacted legislation that funds NORC supportive service programs that require partnerships of housing entities, social services, and health providers to assist older adults to remain living independently in their homes (Amalgamated-Park Reservoir Housing Cooperatives, 2004). NORC supportive service programs can be found in various locations–in big cities, suburbs, and in small towns.

Housing for Older Adults: Senior housing for low-income elders has traditionally included service coordination to prevent institutionalization and to enable older adults to live (semi) independently and interdependently, while providing, as needed, for their basic needs. The U.S. Dept. of Housing and Urban Development (HUD) funds the Section 202 Program for the development of affordable housing for very low income elderly (62 years of age or older). The program in 2004 funded approximately 5,300 units with $495 million. The program also funds project operating costs and residents only pay 30% of their annual income for the housing. The projects are developed by nonprofit organizations and the HUD funding provides a substantial portion of the construction and land acquisition costs, and possibly all the development costs in lower cost areas of the country. The projects must include a supportive services program, which can include a social services coordinator and in-kind services from community resources. Services often include medical screenings, mental health counseling, lectures or classes in nutrition and health issues, recreation opportunities, and exercise classes. Service coordinators provide advocacy for the individual residents needing assistance with social security payments, Medicare, etc. Other services can include meals on wheels and transportation. The projects must also provide services for the frail elderly who are aging in place to prevent the frail elderly being institutionalized and to allow residents to live independently in their home as long as possible.

FIGURE 1 (continued)

Assisted Living Facility (ALF) : Assisted living facilities provide various types of residential living for older adults who require some level of assistance with activities of daily living but do not require nursing home care. More than a million Americans live in an estimated 20,000 assisted/supportive living residences, the fastest growing residential service for older adults (Assisted Living Federation [ALFA], 2004). Assisted living residences provide a combination of housing, personalized supportive services, and health care for elders in need of assistance with activities of daily living. Assisted living facilities vary widely in size, from a few residents to hundreds, and may be owned and operated by not-for-profit or private entities. They typically offer private rooms or small apartments, common areas for socializing and recreation, planned activities, 24-hour staffing, and controlled access. Most assisted living facilities offer support services, including meals served in a common dining area or taken to a resident's room, shuttles for errands and appointments, housekeeping, help with medication management, and emergency call monitoring. Assisted living facilities also offer some resident supervision.

Special Needs Housing: Long in use in the disability and mental health fields, this term generally describes permanent housing targeted to residents of varying ages with a wide range of special needs, including those with mental, developmental, and/or physical disabilities, or who require ongoing treatment and/or attention (e.g., people with HIV/AIDS, people with psychiatric or physical disabilities, and people in recovery from addictions). Services in special needs housing are generally focused on health, mental health, and/or recovery services, in addition to life skills and stabilization services, crisis intervention, and case management. Again, as with many other types of housing linked to services, programs and activities are provided to promote quality of life for residents and to enable them to live both independently and interdependently.

Supportive Housing: The major goal of supportive housing is to prevent homelessness or a recurrence of homelessness through the provision of a comprehensive support system to help residents live independently and interdependently in the community. While supportive housing is most often targeted to individuals who are homeless, formerly homeless, or at risk of homelessness, supportive housing has also been developed for older adults, persons with chronic mental illness, disabled persons, or people in recovery from addictions.

of characteristics (Housing *Plus* Services, 2005b). After much discussion over the perceptions associated with a variety of possible terms, members of the Housing *Plus* Services Committee agreed in 2001 to use *housing plus services* as a general description for housing in which there is a social services connec- tion (Granruth & Smith, 2001).

The Committee also identified general characteristics of *housing plus ser- vices* initiatives, which include the following: (1) the mission of the housing initiative remains broad, i.e., "to enhance quality of life" (although there may be more specific goals identified and programs initiated to achieve these goals, they do not overshadow this general purpose); (2) resident participation in ser- vices is voluntary (excluded are programs whose focus is treatment and resi- dents' participation in services is the reason for admission); and (3) residents, property managers, and service providers work as a team, i.e., there is commu- nication between landlords and residents on the resident's service needs, which may be accomplished through tenant councils, interagency agreements, etc., regarding the operation of the property (Cohen et al., 2004, p. 521). Based on those guidelines, the Housing *Plus* Services Committee then developed a typology and matrix in which the different housing types are identified based on general target population (including older adults), common goals or outcomes, primary services, and general requirement and restrictions.

For this paper, the typology is used to develop the following overview of the basic housing *plus* services settings in which older adults might live independently (or semi-independently) in the community, while at the same time being linked to vital and responsive support systems. These key housing types include *service-enriched housing, public housing, naturally occurring retirement communities, housing for older adults, assisted living facilities, special needs housing,* and *supportive housing.* While the descriptions are at times similar and, in fact, often overlapping, each generally defines a particular type of living arrangement in which a *housing plus services* linkage exists.

As this typology indicates, older adults can be found as residents in a wide range of housing models linked to services. Housing types often share purposes and service delivery strategies. Funding sources for services within housing settings vary considerably and can come from a combination of state and local sources (American Association of Homes and Services for the Aging, 1996), often requiring continuous attention to securing sufficient funds for operation and integrating funding streams.

PRINCIPLES FOR SERVICE DELIVERY IN HOUSING SETTINGS

Given the contemporary challenges and array of service delivery systems in housing settings, the Housing *Plus* Services Committee of the National Low Income Housing Coalition has proposed eleven guiding principles (see Figure 2) for adoption in all permanent housing settings (Housing *Plus* Services, 2005c). These principles were developed through a process of systematic review, consensus building among service providers, and feedback from the larger professional community (Granruth & Smith, 2001). According to Lewis, "the practice principle is the most powerful intellectual tool in a profession's practice" (Lewis, 1982, p. 57). Constructed from values, ethics, practice wisdom, clients' experience, as well as empirically-based knowledge, principles are not simply what is known, but also, what is believed to be important. As the case studies in this paper will demonstrate, we believe that they are of particular utility in housing settings with older adults.

FIGURE 2. Principles for Delivery of Services in Housing Settings (Housing Plus Services, 2005c)

1. Housing is a basic human need, and all people have a right to safe, decent, affordable, and permanent housing.

2. All people are valuable, and capable of being valuable residents and valuable community members.

3. Housing and services should be integrated to enhance the social and economic well-being of residents and to build healthy communities.

4. Residents, owners, property managers, and service providers should work together as a team in integrated housing and services initiatives.

5. Programs should be based on assessments of residents' and community strengths and needs, supported by ongoing monitoring and evaluation.

6. Programs should strengthen and expand resident participation to improve the community's capacity to create change.

7. Residents' participation in programs should be voluntary, with an emphasis on outreach to the most vulnerable.

8. Community development activities should be extended to the neighboring area and residents.

9. Assessment, intervention, and evaluation should be multi-level, focusing on individual resident, groups, and the community.

10. Services should maximize the use of existing resources, avoid duplication, and expand the economic, social, and political resources available to residents.

11. Residents of Housing Plus Services programs should be integrated into the larger community.

Exemplars of Principled Practice

The following case examples are presented from the service providers' perspective to illustrate how principles are put into practice under real life, challenging conditions. Resident names and other distinguishing items have been changed to protect confidentiality. The first two cases are drawn from the work of the New York-based NORC Supportive Program for Seniors, a collaborative effort of the Amalgamated-Park Reservoir Housing Cooperatives, Bronx Jewish Community Council, and the Jewish Home and Hospital Lifecare System. Case one depicts the experience of a couple living in private, regulated rental housing. Case two presents the experience of a woman living in a mixed age, not-for-profit cooperative. Case three is drawn from the experience of the American Association of Homes and Services for the Aging and a white paper entitled *Affordable Assisted Living: Options for Converting or Expanding Housing to Assisted Living–Four*

Case Studies (American Association of Homes and Services to the Aging. 1997), and focuses on two neighbors living in an assisted living residence.

Case One: Charlene and Alfred Charles, Living in Private Rental Housing[1]

Charlene and Alfred Charles live in a privately owned apartment building · in the area. Mrs. Charles is 78 years old, has a thyroid condition and appears to have suffered small strokes. When she was referred to us she had not seen her doctor in over 18 months and not taken any of her medications. This affected her mental health, as she was agitated and often did not make sense. Her husband is 87 years old with obvious signs of dementia. Their clothes were dirty and they appeared not to have bathed. Mr. Charles is a retired civil servant.

The Director of the Senior Center where they had been eating lunch, but had stopped coming, referred the clients to us at NORC. The managing agent of their apartment building contacted the Senior Center Director. The couple had not responded to legal papers they had received, which stated that eviction proceedings would begin if they did not clean their apartment. Neighbors had complained about the condition of the apartment and odors coming into the hallway.

Following the referral, I made several phone calls to introduce myself and to schedule an appointment for a home visit. They were quite hesitant to meet me. They insisted they never received any legal papers. When they finally agreed to see me, they would only see me in the lobby and would not allow me upstairs. They are both hard of hearing, making everything go very slowly. When they finally came to the lobby to see me and we began talking, they accused me of embarrassing them and did not understand why I was interfering. I explained we were trying to help them stay at home and that the danger of eviction was quite real.

When they let me into their apartment, it was quite hazardous. There were piles all over. Stacks of dirty dishes were in the kitchen. There were no safe paths to walk from room to room and the lovely view of the park was totally obstructed. They insisted it would only take 15 minutes to clean and that the managing agent had not sent them anything. To me, it seemed more than likely that the papers were buried in one of their piles.

After case consultation with our staff, it was decided that it was necessary to make a referral to Adult Protective Services, which would most likely order cleaning of the apartment. We worked with Adult Protective Services to arrange for cleaning and to limit their intervention to emergency measures. Once the managing agent learned that the cleaning would be done he cancelled legal proceedings.

We also attempted to help them receive medical attention. They insisted they had a doctor two hours away and he was the only one they trusted. However, they had no way to get to him. After many phone conversations with their doctor, we had their prescriptions renewed and after even more conversations with Mr. and Mrs. Charles they accepted a referral to a local geriatrician. Once they saw the new physician and their medications were stabilized they became more coherent. With their permission, we were able to consult their new doctor, and obtained a greater understanding of their health and what had been happening with them.

At this point, they have resumed their lunches at the Senior Center and Mrs. Charles has even joked about how the first social worker who saw her (me!) was someone who she did not feel too good about. As our work with them continued, they told us about their nephew who is very smart and who would help them. When we reached him, he said he would look to be of assistance and has helped in arranging for home care and personal care for them. They have discussed the possibility of guardianship by the nephew, and have consulted with lawyers who work with us on these issues.

Case Two: Esther Rothman, Living in a Not-For-Profit Cooperative
Housing in a Naturally Occurring Retirement Community[2]

Despite being an urban area, our neighborhood is quite hilly and shady. Particularly in icy or rainy weather, this makes it even more difficult for older people to get around. The only option for shopping within walking distance is a small supermarket. Frequently sighted are elderly people using their shopping carts, not just for shopping but also for support. They will state they are embarrassed to use a walker, and the shopping cart serves that function without the stigma. There are busses within walking distance. There are two subway lines within a 15-20 minute walk. Many seniors are nervous about using the subway. Two local agencies offer shopping trips every other week to a variety of shopping areas and there is also a publicly funded van program for disabled people and a variety of local car services that cost more money.

Esther Rothman is a retired professional woman in her mid 80s who lives in our community. She has multiple medical problems, which impact her mobility. When she was healthier and when her friends were driving and taking public transportation, she was busy attending local concerts, lectures, and community events. However, this has become increasingly difficult. She is a member of our NORC Advisory Board and brought up her concerns about getting around at a monthly meeting.

Our Advisory Board is composed of residents from the various buildings and organizations in our community. The Board has assumed an advocacy role for issues of importance to seniors and is also acting as an eye in the community, alerting us to new clients we might reach. It also brings the management and the social service component together so we are working in unison.

In responding to Mrs. Rothman at the meeting, there was a lot of empathy from the members and further discussion about transportation difficulties. People mentioned other acquaintances that were isolated. Some people who still drive stated how they felt increasingly uncomfortable with the responsibility of giving rides to people who are very weak and who need assistance getting in and out of the car. One typical comment at the meeting was: *there is no point staying in your own home, if you are alone all the time.* Someone else added that at some point they could all be in similar situations and would need this kind of help with transportation. The representative from management acknowledged the reality of this problem.

During the course of discussion, we decided to do an inventory of transportation possibilities (assigned as a project for a student intern). In addition, the idea of dedicating our fundraising efforts to improving transportation options was enthusiastically accepted. When our intern completes the inventory of transportation options in our community, the intern will report back to the Advisory Board who will then seek to develop a comprehensive plan to address this issue. In the short term, the board is making a commitment to help those interested in attending upcoming music classes to obtain transportation. From Esther Rothman raising the issue, we hope to be able to reach a large group of people who share this problem. We see this as a community building effort.

Case Three: Rafael Brown and Angela Murphy, Neighbors in an Assisted Living Facility

Rafael Brown, at 93 years of age, lives in an Elms Residential Community (ERC) which consists of three adjoining HUD Section 202 projects with more than 300 apartments. Next door to him lives Angela Murphy, who is 84. Mr. Brown was and is in notably good health, though he does not cook and never liked to eat alone. Mrs. Murphy has long been confined to a wheelchair and, though she loves to cook, was not always able to prepare meals each and every day. Neither was capable of handling regular housecleaning responsibilities. Both have been active supporters of the resident association, and volunteering at the resident-run Country Store, located on the first floor of the building to provide convenient access to basic food supplies and some additional niceties (handcrafts, toiletries, stationery, etc.). ERC staff provides regular transportation for Country Store volunteers to shop at a bulk foods store every other week, though Mr. Brown has been known to run to the local grocery store to supplement perishable supplies of milk and bread when stock has dwindled too low for comfort.

Both chose to live at ERC because the non-profit, faith-based sponsor initially offered limited activities and a mini-bus for group outings, and a small adult day health center, one meal a day, and a housekeeping program under the auspices of HUD's Congregate Housing Services Program (CHSP). Mr. Brown and Mrs. Murphy developed a close friendship, stemming from the loss of their respective partners just before moving in, and helped each other with a range of informal supportive services. Particularly notable, they always shared their meals–whether prepared by Mrs. Murphy, or as part of the CHSP program. Their interdependence helped both immensely, but lately their need for formalized services increased.

With Mrs. Murphy's rapidly advancing degenerative condition, she could no longer independently dress herself and was having increasing difficulty preparing food and sometimes even feeding herself. Mr. Brown began to have trouble keeping track of his bills, and required some assistance where money-management was involved. Both recognized the need for more extensive help in meal preparation and other basic activities of daily living.

With the average age of new admissions rising from 60 to older than 75, and an average age of residents near 80, ERC had been proactively developing an ever-increasing array of services initiatives. By the time Mr. Brown and Mrs. Murphy needed more assistance, ERC had developed a large adult day health center, a small social day care program, initiated a wheelchair accessible van service for residents and day center clients, and increased their staffing to include a full-time activities director and a HUD supportive services coordinator.

DISCUSSION OF IMPLEMENTATION OF PRINCIPLES

These exemplary case studies illustrate challenges to putting the principles proposed by the National Low Income Housing Coalition into practice, as well as successes in integrating the principles into work with older adults and their communities. Each case highlights difficulties in living and the interface of the individual residents with their environment. They also demonstrate how effective, evolving services can facilitate this interface, helping older adults to remain in their homes while maintaining as much control over their lives as possible. At the same time, they portray older adults as contributors to community life, and as people with strengths as well as difficulties.

When encroachments on self-determination must be made, as in the second case study where eviction was imminent, it is done thoughtfully, and limited to emergency areas that represent a danger to self and others. Services should not reinforce losses but rather create environments where self-determination is supported. Of course, service providers must intervene when there is a severe threat to the life of residents, but in most situations residents should not be forced to participate in service, and their refusals should be honored. Before imposing any mandatory elements in service delivery, providers must ask themselves if such action is truly needed, and if voluntary options have been fully explored. Thus, the principles are consistent with the recommendations of the United States Commission on Affordable Housing and Health Facility Needs for Seniors in the 21st Century (2002), which suggests that services for older adults be built on the interrelated values of dignity, security and independence.

In the first case, Mr. and Mrs. Charles attended the local senior center, the first program to become aware of their situation. In the second, Mrs. Rothman was an active member of the NORC Advisory Committee. Mr. Brown and Mrs. Murphy of the third case formed a strong support system and also volunteered at the Country Store. These connections were strengthened through the provision of services, and indicate that helping to maintain the web of social relationships is an important objective of services in housing settings. Older adults report that relationships between friends and peers are critically important as "they experience the eroding capabilities and negative feedback that contradict their identity perceptions" (Siebert, Mutran, & Reitzes, 1999, p. 530). Therefore, services should foster reciprocal relationships of mutual assistance, in which each participant both gives and receives support and assistance.

As modeled by the service providers in these case studies, workers providing services in housing settings should be able to move among a variety of roles, including those of facilitator, educator, researcher, mediator, advocate, consultant, and convener. Service providers act as a bridge to the larger community by becoming known to outside agencies, engaging in reciprocal arrangements, and encouraging resident participation in broader venues. This need for flexibility is extended to the service delivery system itself, which must engage in continual assessment and ongoing development to meet evolving needs of residents.

The older residents, owners/property managers, and service providers worked together to address the difficulties raised in these case studies, reinforcing the lesson of strong community collaboration, and participation by all community constituents. Successful housing programs have demonstrated the efficacy of engaging residents directly in the process of community change (Reynolds & Hamburger, 1997; Tull, 1999) and building social capital (Saegert & Winkel, 1998). Each story included a range of responses to individual concerns, and problems were addressed on an individual, family, small group, and community-wide level. The experience of service delivery affirmed the participants' sense of themselves as contributors.

In the three case studies, multiple sources of resources were engaged, including from peers, social service providers, family members, and other neighbors. All constituent groups in housing settings should understand and respect one another's role and functions, and subscribe to a common mission of building a successful community. Managers must be concerned with the welfare of tenants, while service providers must be concerned with obstacles that prevent continued occupancy (Cohen & Phillips, 1997). This collective consciousness must also extend to the residents, who work in partnership with staff and owners/housing developers.

All three cases also point out the changing needs of residents as they age, and how what was once a satisfactory housing arrangement can rapidly shift to a place of barriers and difficulties. As the residents' issues were assessed, the most immediate problems were addressed quickly, in some cases with direct action (such as involvement of Adult Protective Services to avoid eviction of Mr. and Mrs. Charles) and in other cases, through support and more modest interventions (such as mutual support and immediate transportation options for Mrs. Rothman and her neighbors, and food service and personal care for Mr. Brown and Mrs. Murphy). In different circumstances, it is possible that all of them might have had to move into a nursing home or other more service-rich environment. Instead, the integration of services in these housing settings led to continued independence coupled with greater connection.

These cases have been presented to demonstrate how service providers ideally provide options and choices, rather than prescriptions (Shafer, 2001). In this spirit, the eleven principles serve to inform and unify practice without determinism. Across type of housing setting, communities, and funding streams, the core principles allow for a wide range of best practices to emerge, linked to the particular challenges and strengths of diverse environments.

CONCLUSION

A sense of *home* is one of the most enduring images in our collective psyche. Whether it is the *home sweet home* of the folk art sampler or *a place to call home* of more recent vintage, we like to think of home as a secure, nourishing place of permanence (Hirsch, Kett, & Trefil, 2002). The need for home crosses age and life condition. In spite of this, for many home is not a refuge, but rather a source of difficulty and insecurity. Housing is at the social, economic, and political center of community life (Millennial Housing Commission, 2002). By linking services with housing, we can have an impact in all of these spheres. Services integrated with housing provide a stabilizing force to keep buildings safe and secure and to foster a critical sense of community.

It has been the position of this paper that principle-guided practice is essential in delivering services to older adults and all residents across a range of housing settings. For Charlene and Alfred Charles, Esther Rothman, and Rafael Brown and Angela Murphy, effective services made the difference between *home sweet home* and *leaving home*. We believe that the adoption of these core principles will enable many more vulnerable elders to enjoy the benefits of aging-in-place, instead of having to face the likelihood of unnecessary displacement and/or institutionalization. With integrated services, older residents will continue to bring their skills to the ongoing work of community building in the places they call home.

NOTES

1. This couple resides in privately owned, rent regulated housing in a community identified as a Naturally Occurring Retirement Community (NORC) served by a state-funded, not-for-profit service program. For another case study of an older adult living in housing owned by a not-for-profit corporation, see Cohen et al. (2004).

2. Residents in this case study reside in a 75 year old, not-for-profit cooperative housing community for people of all ages founded by the Amalgamated Clothing Workers Union, which has been designated a Naturally Occurring Retirement Community (NORC).

REFERENCES

Amalgamated-Park Reservoir Housing Cooperatives. (2004). NORC: *Supportive program for seniors*. New York: Amalgamated-Park Reservoir Housing Cooperatives.

American Association of Homes and Services for the Aging (AAHSA). (1997). *Affordable assisted living: Options for converting or expanding housing to assisted living: Four case studies*. Washington, DC: American Association of Homes and Services for the Aging.

American Association of Homes and Services to the Aging (AAHSA). (1996). *Integrated funding streams: A discussion paper*. Washington, DC: American Association of Homes and Services to the Aging.

Americans with Disability Act of 1990, P.L. 101-336, 104 Stat. 327.

Assisted Living Federation of America (ALFA). (2004). *What is assisted living?* Available online at: *http://www.alfa.org*.

Beattie, B., Whitelaw, N., Mettler, M., & Turner, D. (2003). A vision of older adults and health promotion. *American Journal of Health Promotion, 18*(2), 200-204.

Blieszner, R. (1986). Trends in family gerontology research. *Family Relations, 35*, 555-562.

Caplan, G., Williams, A., Daly, B., & Abraham, K. (2004). A randomized controlled trial of comprehensive geriatric assessment and multidisciplinary intervention after discharge of elderly from the emergency department–the DEED II study. *Journal of the American Geriatrics Society, 52*(9), 1417-1423.

Challis, D., Darton, R., Hughes, J., Stewart, K., & Weiner, K. (2001). Intensive care management at home: An alternative to institutional care? *Age and Ageing, 30,* 409-413.

Cohen, C. S., Mulroy, E., Tull, T., White, C., & Crowley, S. (2004). Housing plus services: Supporting vulnerable families in permanent housing. *Child Welfare, LXXXIII*(5), 509-528.

Cohen, C. S., & Phillips, M. (1997). Building community: Principles for social work practice in housing settings. *Social Work, 42,* 471-481.

Dear, M., & Wolch, J. (1979). The optimal assignment of human service clients to treatment settings (pp.197-210). In S. Golant (Ed.). *Location and Environment of Elderly Population.* Washington, DC: V.H. Winston & Sons.

Golant, S. (2003). Political and organizational barriers to satisfying low-income U.S. seniors' need for affordable rental housing with supportive services. *Journal of Aging & Social Policy, 15*(4), 21-48.

Golant, S. (1984). *A Place to Grow Old: The Meaning of Environment in Old Age.* New York: Columbia University Press.

Governor's Conference on Aging. (2004). *Aging 2020 Summit.* Phoenix: Arizona Governor's Office.

Granruth, L. B., & Smith, C. H. (2001). *Low income housing and service programs: Towards a new perspective.* Washington, DC: National Low Income Housing Coalition.

Grimmer, K. A., Moss, J. R., & Gill, T. K. (2000). Discharge planning quality from the career perspective. *Quality of Life Research, 9,* 1005-1013.

Hirsch, E. D., Kett, J. F., & Trefil, J. (2002). *The new dictionary of cultural literacy.* Boston: Houghton Mifflin Company.

Housing *Plus* Services Committee of the National Low Income Housing Coalition. (2005a). *http://www.housingplusservices.org/.* Washington, DC: National Low Income Housing Coalition.

Housing *Plus* Services Committee of the National Low Income Housing Coalition. (2005b). *http://www.housingplusservices.org/typology.pdf.* Washington, DC: National Low Income Housing Coalition.

Housing *Plus* Services Committee of the National Low Income Housing Coalition. (2005c). *http://www.housingplusservices.org/principles.pdf.* Washington, DC: National Low Income Housing Coalition.

Ivry, J. (1995). Aging in place: The role of geriatric social work. *Families in Society, Feb.,* 76-85.

Kornblatt, S., Cheng, S., & Chan, S. (2002). Best practice: The On Lok model of geriatric interdisciplinary team care. *Journal of Gerontological Social Work, 40*(1/2), 15-22.

Lewis, H. (1982). *The intellectual base of social work practice.* Binghamton, NY: Haworth Press.

Linzer, N. (2002). An ethical dilemma in home care. *Journal of Gerontological Social Work, 37*(2), 22-34.

Logan, R., & Applebaum, R. (1995). Funding elder home care from the bottom up: Policy choices for a local community. *Generations*, Fall, *19*(3), 75-77.

Millennial Housing Commission. (2002). *Meeting Our Nation's Housing Challenges.* Washington, DC: U.S. Government Printing Office.

Mollica, R. (2003). Coordinating services across the continuum of health, housing, and supportive services. *Journal of Aging and Health, 15*(1), 165-188.

Mulroy, E. (2003). Community as a factor in implementing interorganizational partnerships: Issues, constraints, and adaptations. *Nonprofit Management and Leadership, 14*(1), 47-66.

Mutchler, J. E., & Burr, J. A. (2003). Living arrangements among older persons. *Research on Aging, 25*(6), 531-558.

National Low Income Housing Coalition (NLIHC). (2005). Annual Housing Policy Conference and Lobby Day. *http://www.nlihc.org/conference.pdf.* Washington, DC: National Low Income Housing Coalition.

Pine, P., & Pine, V. R. (2002). Naturally occurring retirement community-supportive service program: An example of devolution. *Journal of Aging & Social Policy, 14*(3/4), 181-193.

Pynoos, J., & Liebig, P. (1995). Housing policy for frail elders: Trends and implications for long term care. In J. Pynoos, & P. Liebig (Eds.). *Housing frail elders: International policies, perspectives, and prospects.* Baltimore: Johns Hopkins University Press.

Pynoos, J., & Nishita, C. M. (2003). The cost and financing of home modifications in the United States. *Journal of Disability Policy Studies, 14*(2), 68-73.

Pynoos, J., & Regnier, V. (1991). Improving residential environments for frail elderly: Bridging the gap between theory and application. In J. Birren, J. Lubben, J. Rowe, & D. Deutchman (Eds.). *The Concept and Measurement of Quality of Life in the Frail Elderly* (pp. 91-119). New York: Academic Press.

Reynolds, S., & Hamburger, S. (1997). *Not a solo act: Creating successful partnerships to develop and operate supportive housing.* New York: Corporation for Supportive Housing.

Runciman, P., Currie, C. T., Nicol, M., Green, L., & McKay, V. (1996). Discharge of elderly people from an accident and emergency department: Evaluation of health visitor follow up. *Journal of Advanced Nursing, 24*, 711-718.

Saegert, S., & Winkel, G. (1998). Social capital and revitalization of New York City's distressed housing. *Housing Policy Debate, 9*(1) 17-60.

Shafer, D. N. (2001). Service coordinators' key to success. *Journal of Housing & Community Development. 58*(3) 36.

Siebert, D. C., Mutran, E. J., & Reitzes, D. C. (1999). Friendship and social support: The importance of role identity to aging adults. *Social Work, 44*(6) 522-533.

Stewart, S. (2003). "A Tapestry of Voices": Using Elder Focus Groups to Guide Applied Research Practice. *Journal of Gerontological Social Work*, Vol. 42(1), pg. 77-88.

Struyk, R., Page, D. B., Newman, S., Carroll, M., Ueno, M., Cohen, B., & Wright, P. (1989). *Providing supportive services to the frail elderly in federally assisted housing.* Urban Institute Report 89-2. Washington, DC: Urban Institute Press.

Toseland, R. W., McCallion, P., Gerber, T., Dawson, C., Gieryic, S., & Guilamo-Ramos, V. (1999). Use of health and human services by community-residing people with dementia. *Social Work*, *44*(6), 535-548.

Tull, T. (1999). *Service-enriched housing: Models and methodologies* (Revised edition) Los Angeles: Beyond Shelter.

United States Commission on Affordable Housing and Health Facility Needs for Seniors in the 21st Century. (2002). *A quiet crisis in America: A report to congress.* Washington, DC: U.S. Government Printing Office.

Van der Bij, A. K., Laurant, M. G. H., & Wensing, M. (2002). Effectiveness of physical activity interventions for older adults. *American Journal of Preventive Medicine*, *22*(2), 120-133.

Yeates, M. (1979). The need for environmental perspectives on issues facing older people. In S. Golant (Ed.). *Location and Environment of Elderly Population* (pp. 71-80). Washington, DC: V.H. Winston & Sons.

doi:10.1300/J083v49n01_09

Anticipating Relocation:
Concerns About Moving
Among NORC Residents

Brian D. Carpenter, PhD
Dorothy F. Edwards, PhD
Joseph G. Pickard, MSW
Janice L. Palmer, RN, MS
Susan Stark, PhD, OTR/L
Peggy S. Neufeld, PhD, OTR/L
Nancy Morrow-Howell, PhD
Margaret A. Perkinson, PhD
John C. Morris, MD

Support for this project was provided by the Administration on Aging (90AM2612) and the State of Missouri in grants to the Jewish Federation of St. Louis, by the Harvey A. and Dorismae Friedman Research Fund at Washington University in St. Louis, and by the Washington University Center for Aging. This study was facilitated by the Jewish Federation of St. Louis Naturally Occurring Retirement Community (NORC) team under the direction of Dr. Stephen Cohen and Coordinator Karen Berry Elbert, who provided logistical support during the recruitment and data collection process. Many undergraduate and graduate students in the departments of Occupational Therapy, Psychology, and Social Work conducted in-home interviews. The authors also wish to acknowledge the gracious contribution made by all the participants in inviting interviewers into their homes and sharing their thoughts and concerns. Finally, two anonymous reviewers provided thoughtful comments that helped clarify the presentation and interpretation of our findings.

[Haworth co-indexing entry note]: "Anticipating Relocation: Concerns About Moving Among NORC Residents." Carpenter, Brian D. et al. Co-published simultaneously in *Journal of Gerontological Social Work* (The Haworth Press, Inc.) Vol. 49, No. 1/2, 2007, pp. 165-184; and: *Housing for the Elderly: Policy and Practice Issues* (ed: Philip McCallion) The Haworth Press, Inc., 2007, pp. 165-184. Single or multiple copies of this article are available for a fee from The Haworth Document Delivery Service [1-800-HAWORTH, 9:00 a.m. - 5:00 p.m. (EST). E-mail address: docdelivery@haworthpress.com].

SUMMARY. Most older adults prefer to live at home as long as possible, requiring supports and services to help them age in place. This study examines the relocation concerns of a group of older adults in a suburban naturally-occurring retirement community (NORC). Twenty-six percent of the 324 residents interviewed expressed concern about having to move in the next few years. Residents who were worried differed from those who did not worry on a number of demographic and biopsychosocial characteristics. Overall, residents present a profile of vulnerability that calls for preemptive action to help them stay in their homes. A NORC is an ideal setting in which to provide supportive services. doi:10.1300/J083v49n01_10 *[Article copies available for a fee from The Haworth Document Delivery Service: 1-800-HAWORTH. E-mail address: <docdelivery@haworthpress.com> Website: <http:// www.HaworthPress.com> © 2007 by The Haworth Press, Inc. All rights reserved.]*

KEYWORDS. Housing, relocation, NORC

ANTICIPATING RELOCATION: CONCERNS ABOUT MOVING AMONG NORC RESIDENTS

Recent policy and service initiatives strive to help older adults remain in their current homes as long as possible, reflecting the many advantages of "aging in place." Older adults prefer to stay in their own homes (AARP, 2000; Glassman, 1998), or at least to stay in the same neighborhood if relocation becomes necessary (Groves & Wilson, 1992). Indeed, some types of relocations can have deleterious consequences on health, at least in the short term (Lutgendorf et al., 2001). And, the costs of helping older adults stay at home can be significantly less than those associated with residential care (Lawler, 2001), at least for some individual households.

Nonetheless, each year a significant number of older adults do relocate. Some move by choice, to be in a warmer climate or closer to relatives or friends. For other older adults, however, it may be inaccurate to say that they *choose* to move, as the distinction between a voluntary and involuntary move is often clouded by circumstance. For instance, following divorce (Booth & Amato, 1990) or widowhood (Chevan, 1995), an older adult may relocate in response to a change in financial resources or a realignment of social network. Should this be considered a voluntary move? Similarly, changes in physical health and functional ability, such as those following a stroke or hip fracture, might prompt relocation if an older adult requires a living environment with more support and supervision (Wiseman, 1980). Here again, an older adult may decide she needs to live somewhere else, but the decision is propelled by circumstances beyond the individual's control. In sum, relocations result from a complex interplay of personal and situational factors that are highly individualistic and not always obviously voluntary or involuntary.

One useful model for understanding relocation among older adults has been presented by Litwak and Longino (1987). Taking a lifespan developmental perspective, they argue that older adults are likely to experience three basic types of moves late in life. The first occurs postretirement and is motivated by amenities and lifestyle choices (e.g., migrating to Florida). The second occurs when chronic disabilities limit the accomplishment of everyday tasks; this type of move often involves relocating to be closer to children or other kin who can help with care. The third type of move occurs when kin are no longer able to provide the level of support that is needed and institutional care is required.

The implication of this model and others (e.g., Wiseman, 1980) is that there are both risk factors and protective factors associated with late-life relocations. Previous research with older adults after they have moved has identified three primary factors associated with relocation: physical health, social network, and financial status. Using a retrospective method, relocations seem most often prompted by an increase in chronic health conditions (Brown, Liang, Krause, Akiyama, Sugisawa, & Fukaya, 2002), a decline in functional independence (Colsher & Wallace, 1990), and an overall deterioration in physical health (Gardner, 1994). So too are moves likely to occur when older adults are living alone (Miller & Weissert, 2000), with an insufficient informal caregiving network nearby (Forbes, Hoffart, & Redford, 1997; Johnson, Schwiebert, & Rosenmann, 1994). Lastly, older adults with lower income (Colsher & Wallace, 1990) who face increasing costs associated with their housing (O'Bryant & Murray, 1987) and those who rent rather than own their homes (Miller & Weissert, 2000) appear vulnerable to relocation.

As a group, these studies identified causes of relocation after the fact, pinpointing triggering events or circumstances that incited a move. In the current study, by contrast, we were interested in taking a prospective approach and asking older adults whether they felt vulnerable regarding future relocation and, if so, why. Identifying risk factors for relocation may enable service providers to preempt a move that could be avoided.

Another unique feature of this study is that we approached older adults living in a suburban naturally-occurring retirement community (NORC). The operational definition of a NORC has evolved over the years (see Callahan & Lanspery, 1997) and communities thought of as NORCs are diverse in terms of location, physical and geographic dimensions, population and demographic characteristics, ownership patterns, and available service networks. Some NORCs consist of older adults living in one apartment building, while others reflect a neighborhood or even small town (Hunt, 2001). NORCs also come into existence for a variety of reasons: some arise when older adults move into a neighborhood, others emerge when citizens who have lived for some time in a building or area "age in place" together, and still others are created by both processes simultaneously. In all their forms, however, NORCs are characterized by a disproportionate number of older residents. Older adults congregate in these locations for practical, psychological, and social reasons; the places provide what they need in order to live independent, fulfilling lives as they grow older.

We were interested in studying what we refer to as *anticipatory relocation* among these suburban NORC residents for two interrelated reasons. First, the large concentration of older adults in this neighborhood provide access to a sample of individuals who are heterogeneous in their individual needs yet relatively homogeneous in terms of their access to neighborhood facilities and services. Second, once relocation risk factors have been identified, the NORC itself presents an economy of scale for developing supportive interventions to help older adults age in place in their homes. The suburban NORC we studied included a geographic region that had a disproportionate number of residents over age 60, based on current census data (U.S. Census Bureau, 2000). Residents within this NORC either aged in place (i.e., they had been living in post-WWII tract homes in this suburb for many years) or had migrated to the area to live in apartments, condominiums, or congregate housing surrounded by a neighborhood network of aging services.

To summarize the study, we compared older adults who worried that they would need to move in the near future to older adults who expressed no such concern. Our goal was to identify resident characteristics associated with vulnerability to relocation.

METHODS

Participants and Procedure

Participants were drawn from a geographically-defined, naturally-occurring retirement community approximately one square mile in size in the St. Louis suburbs. The boundaries of the NORC were based on a circumscribed set of apartment buildings, townhouse apartments, condominiums, single-family homes, senior congregate housing facilities, and the business and service organizations that sprang up around them as, historically, more and more older adults moved into this neighborhood. According to the U.S. Census Bureau (2000), this NORC neighborhood includes 4,641 residents, of whom 47% (2,172) are age 50 or older, and 32% (1,487) are age 65 or older. The percentage of residents age 65 and older is substantially higher than in the county and state as a whole (14% and 13%, respectively).

Between January 2003, and October 2003, adults over age 65 in the NORC who had responded to initial recruitment efforts by the research team were invited to participate in an interview regarding their service needs, service use, and preferences. Recruitment efforts included door-to-door solicitation; media outlets including newspaper, radio, and television; booths at health fairs and local grocery stores; presentations to community, church, and tenant groups; and direct mailings. Potential participants were screened by phone to ensure that they met the residency and age requirements and were willing to participate in a 2-hour, in-home interview. The interviews were conducted by members of the research team and undergraduate and graduate student research assistants who had completed an intensive training program. Interviews included a broad range of biopsychosocial assessments, a portion of which are described in this report. At the conclusion of the interview, participants were debriefed, paid $20, and invited to make their name available for additional projects. A total of 324 participants completed the in-home interview.

Measures

Demographic Characteristics

Basic demographic data collected included age, gender, marital status, whether the resident was currently living alone, race/ethnicity, years of education, and household income. Respondents also indicated whether their residence was a single-family home, condominium, apartment, or congregate housing; and whether they owned their home, were paying a mortgage, or paid rent. An additional question about *subjective financial security* read, "Financially, how hard is it to make ends meet?" Responses were made on a 5-point Likert-type scale ranging from *very easy* (1) to *very hard* (5).

Physical health. Self-rated health was assessed with the question, "In general, would you say your health is . . . ." Responses ranged from *poor* (1) to *excellent* (5). *Number of chronic conditions* was assessed with the 27-item Cornell Medical Index Health Questionnaire (Brodman, Erdmann, & Wolf, 1960), a checklist of common ailments, such as arthritis, hypertension, and diabetes, as well as more diffuse syndromes such as muscle aches and back pain. The 6-item Blessed Orientation-Memory-Concentration Test (BOMC) (Katzman, Brown, Fuld, Peck, Schechter, & Schimmel, 1983) was used to assess degree of *cognitive impairment*, with higher scores indicating more advanced impairment.

Number of prescription medications was ascertained with the question, "How many prescription drugs do you take?"

Functional capacity. Functional capacity was assessed with two scales from the Duke Older Americans Resources and Services (OARS) survey (Fillenbaum, 1988). A 7-item scale to measure *activities of daily living* (alpha = .72) included items regarding eating, bathing, and basic self-care. A 6-item scale to measure *instrumental activities of daily living* (alpha = .81) included items regarding meal preparation, shopping, and more complex daily activities. Most items were assessed with a 3-point Likert-type scale ranging from *completely unable to perform the task* (0) to *can complete the task without help* (2). Ratings on individual items were summed to yield a total Activities of Daily Living (ADL) score and a total Instrumental Activities of Daily Living (IADL) score, and higher scores indicate greater functional independence.

Social resources. An interviewer-rated assessment of overall current social resources was obtained with the OARS Social Resources Rating Scale Total Score (Fillenbaum, 1988). The interviewer used answers to 9 questions (e.g., frequency of social contacts, presence of a confidant, and subjective perception of available assistance) as a basis for a summary rating on a 6-point Likert-type scale ranging from *excellent social resources* (1) to *totally socially impaired* (6). *Number of informal* helpers was determined by asking residents whether they had people available to help them in case of need. Dichotomous responses (yes/no) to ten categories of relationships were summed to yield a total number of subjective supports. One question about *loneliness* asked, "Do you find yourself feeling lonely?" Response options included *quite often* (0), *sometimes* (1), and *almost never* (2).

Emotional resources. Life satisfaction was assessed with the question, "Taking all things together, how would you say you find life these days?" Responses were made on a 4-point Likert-type scale ranging from *not satisfying* (1) to *very satisfying* (4). The short form of the Geriatric Depression Scale (Lesher & Berryhill, 1994) was used to assess *depressive symptoms*. Fifteen Yes/No items yielded a total depression score (alpha = .79), with higher scores indicating more depressive symptoms. *Recent stress* was ascertained with the question, "How would you rate the average degree of stress that you have experienced during the past 6 months?" Ratings were made on a 10-point scale ranging from *no stress* (1) to *severe stress* (10).

Worry about moving. Participants were asked whether they had concerns about having to move with a question from the Plainview-Old Bethpage Cares Community-Wide Survey (Greenbaum, Kahler, & Finkelstein, 2002): "Do you worry that you will have to move out of your current home within a few years?" Participants responded Yes/No. "Yes" responses were followed by an open-ended question, "Why might you have to move?" Open-ended responses were transcribed verbatim.

Data Analysis

A series of chi-square analyses and *t*-tests were conducted to compare the worried and not worried groups on demographic characteristics, health and functional capacity, social resources, and emotional resources. A multivariate examination of factors that might predict which residents were worried was conducted with a logistic regression. An iterative stepwise approach was used to generate a parsimonious model in which the number of predictor variables was consistent with the overall sample size (Wright, 1995). The dichotomous variable of worried versus not worried was the dependent variable. Step 1 included the demographic variables age, gender, marital status, housing type (dichotomized so that apartment dwelling was the reference group), and subjective financial security. Step 2 included health and functional capacity variables: self-rated health, number of chronic conditions, ADL score, and IADL score. Step 3 included the OARS Social Resources summary score, number of informal helpers, loneliness rating, life satisfaction, Geriatric Depression Scale, and stress rating.

For analysis of qualitative responses to the relocation question, two investigators developed content categories during an initial review of the open-ended responses. They then compared categories and developed a single coding system. Next each investigator coded each concern that was mentioned. Inter-rater reliability for the coding was 91%. Any remaining discrepancies were resolved during a consensus conference.

RESULTS

Eighty-four residents (26%) said they were worried they might have to move in the next few years. Examining why residents feared they might have to move, the majority (65%) expressed concerns about potential health problems that might limit their ability to stay at home (see Figure 1). Next most common were financial concerns (26%), such as the ability to pay rent or condominium fees, particularly were they to increase. A number of residents (12%) felt that architectural features of their residence, such as a large number of stairs or structural features of the bathroom, might force them to move. A few residents expressed concern about being able to maintain their house (6%) given its size. Others said that moving would enable them to stay closer to friends or family, and they feared social isolation if they stayed in their current home (6%). Some residents made a general comment about their own aging

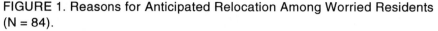

FIGURE 1. Reasons for Anticipated Relocation Among Worried Residents (N = 84).

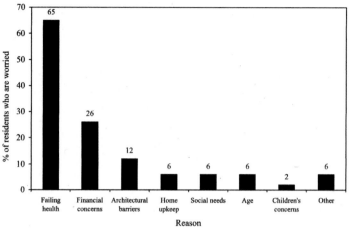

(6%), which seemed to reflect a concern about declining independence and autonomy. Two residents reported that they were being pressured to move by their children, who had concerns about their parents' safety. Other miscellaneous reasons (6%) included worries such as the potential closing of an apartment building and the wishes of a spouse.

Demographic characteristics of the sample appear in Table 1. In initial univariate analyses, the two groups differed on a number of these demographic characteristics. First, a higher proportion of women reported being worried about relocation relative to men (30% versus 17%, $\chi^2(1) = 5.47$, $p < .05$). Likewise, a higher proportion of respondents not currently married were worried about relocation relative to those who were married (31% versus 16%, $\chi^2(1) = 9.13$, $p < .01$). Individuals living in a home, condominium, or congregate senior housing were less likely to be worried about relocation than those living in an apartment, $\chi^2(1) = .24.89$, $p < .001$. And more residents living alone were worried about moving compared to those living with someone else (31% versus 19%, $\chi^2(1) = 5.36$, $p < .05$). Finally, respondents who were worried about relocating were, on average, older than respondents not worried (*M* age = 81.14 years versus 77.66 years, $t(322) = -4.00$, $p < .001$). No group differences were found in race or education.

We had anticipated that people worried about moving would have lower incomes, but we found no significant group differences on this attribute. We might point out that very few of the participants who were worried (2%) were in the upper end of the income range (annual income above $50,000), compared to a higher percentage of those who were not worried (13%). In contrast,

TABLE 1. Sociodemographic Characteristics of the Sample and Tests of Group Differences

Characteristic	Entire sample		Worried (*n* = 84)		Not worried (*n* = 240)	
	n	%	*n*	%	*n*	%
Gender*[a]						
Female	230	71%	68	30%	162	70%
Male	94	29%	16	17%	77	83%
Marital status**						
Married	109	34%	17	16%	92	84%
Not married	215	66%	67	31%	148	69%
Living alone						
Yes	193	60%	59	31%	134	69%
No	131	40%	25	19%	106	81%
Housing type***						
House	40	12%	11	28%	29	72%
Condo	164	51%	42	26%	122	74%
Apartment	51	16%	25	49%	26	51%
Congregate	69	21%	6	9%	63	91%
Race						
Non-white	16	5%	6	36%	10	63%
White	304	95%	78	25%	230	75%
	M	*SD*	*M*	*SD*	*M*	*SD*
Age (yrs)***	78.56	7.04	81.14	6.33	77.66	7.06
Education (yrs)	13.44	2.42	13.23	2.46	13.51	2.40
Income	$24,352	$18,045	$21,726	$13,669	$25,270	$19,285
Subjective financial security[b]***	2.52	0.97	2.90	1.06	2.38	0.90

Note. Percentages for the whole sample represent distribution within the variable, while percentages for the worried and not worried columns represent distribution between groups.
[a] Statistically significant differences between the worried and not worried groups are designated as follows: * $p < .05$, ** $p < .01$, *** $p < .001$.
[b] Higher scores indicate less security about finances.

when asked about subjective financial security (higher scores indicate more financial concerns), those who were worried about moving felt less financially secure (*M* = 2.90, *SD* = 1.06) relative to those not worried about moving (*M* = 2.38, *SD* = 0.90, *t*(319) = −4.35, *p* < .001).

Comparisons regarding the physical health and functional capacity of the worried and not worried residents appear in Table 2. Ratings of overall self-rated health were more negative for the worried residents (*M* = 2.63) relative to the not worried residents (*M* = 3.33, *t*(322) = 5.32, *p* < .001). Likewise, the number of self-reported chronic conditions was higher among worried residents (*M* = 6.57) compared to not worried residents (*M* = 4.69, *t*(319) = −5.47, *p* < .001). Specific

TABLE 2. Health and Functional Capacity, Worried and Not Worried Residents

Variable	Worried ($n = 84$)		Not worried ($n = 240$)	
	M	SD	M	SD
Health				
Self-rated health***[a]	2.63	1.01	3.33	1.04
Number of chronic conditions***	6.57	2.98	4.69	2.58
Short Blessed Test	2.40	3.77	2.23	2.90
Number of prescriptions meds*	4.83	2.85	4.01	3.15
Functional capacity				
ADL score**	13.04	1.50	13.51	0.97
IADL score**	10.47	2.20	11.13	1.68

Note. Higher scores indicate better self-rated health, more chronic conditions, more cognitive impairment, more medications, and greater functional independence.
[a] Significant differences between the worried and not worried are designated as follows: * $p < .05$, ** $p < .01$, *** $p < .001$.

conditions that were more common among worried residents included arthritis, $\chi^2 = 4.75$, $p < .05$; back problems, $\chi^2 = 17.96$, $p < .001$; muscle aches, $\chi^2 = 14.16$, $p < .001$; circulation problems, $\chi^2 = 13.75$, $p < .001$; and urinary disorders, $\chi^2 = 8.14$, $p < .01$. Residents worried about moving also were taking more prescription medications ($M = 4.83$) relative to residents not worried about moving ($M = 4.01$, $t(312) = -2.07$, $p < .05$). No significant differences were found between the two groups in terms of cognitive status, although the BOMC may not be sensitive to very mild impairments in cognition. Regarding functional capacity, worried residents reported slightly more impairment in activities of daily living (lower scores reflect more impairment; $M = 13.04$) than the not worried residents ($M = 13.51$, $t(320) = 3.25$, $p < .01$). Finally, worried residents reported slightly more impairment in instrumental activities of daily living ($M = 10.47$) than not worried residents ($M = 11.13$, $t(320) = 2.82$, $p < .01$).

Comparisons regarding the social and emotional resources of the worried and not worried residents appear in Table 3. Ratings on the OARS Social Resources Rating Scale total score indicated weak social integration and less available support among worried residents (lower scores reflect better resources; $M = 5.05$) relative to not worried residents ($M = 4.30$, $t(318) = 5.03$, $p < .001$). Consistent with this interviewer-assigned rating, residents who were worried said they had fewer informal caregivers ($M = 2.56$) who might be able to provide assistance with activities of daily living, compared to residents who were not worried ($M = 3.47$, $t(322) = 3.41$, $p < .01$). Contrary to expectations, feelings of loneliness were more common among residents who were not worried

TABLE 3. Social and Emotional Resources, Worried and Not Worried Residents

Variable	Worried (n = 84)		Not worried (n = 240)	
	M	SD	M	SD
Social resources				
OARS social resources*** a	4.30	1.30	5.05	1.13
# informal helpers**	2.56	2.00	3.47	2.13
Often feels lonely***	1.00	0.73	1.51	0.63
Emotional resources				
Life satisfaction***	2.55	0.85	3.13	0.76
GDS***	3.78	3.08	2.04	2.35
Recent stress**	5.40	2.07	4.39	2.38

Note. Higher scores indicate better social resources, more informal helpers, more loneliness and greater life satisfaction, more depression and stress.
a Significant differences between the worried and not worried are designated as follows: * $p < .05$, ** $p < .01$, *** $p < .001$.

about relocation ($M = 1.51$) compared to residents worried about relocation ($M = 1.00$, $t(321) = 6.15$, $p < .001$). Nonetheless, residents who were worried about relocation expressed lower overall satisfaction with their lives ($M = 2.55$) compared to residents not worried about moving ($M = 3.13$, $t(320) = 5.78$, $p < .001$). They also endorsed more depressive symptoms ($M = 3.78$ versus $M = 2.04$, $t(320) = -5.34$, $p < .01$) and greater levels of stress in the last 6 months ($M = 5.40$ versus $M = 4.39$, $t(319) = -3.43$, $p < .01$).

In the multivariate logistic regression to identify a set of predictors that might differentiate worried residents from unworried residents, the omnibus test of the coefficient was significant, $\chi 2(5) = 72.37$, $p < .001$, $= 277.38$. Model coefficients, standard errors, and test statistics appear in Table 4. In the final step, the variables that, as a group, were significantly associated with being worried about relocation included older age, apartment dwelling (compared to residents in homes, condominiums, or congregate housing), more concern about financial security, more chronic conditions, and lower life satisfaction. Variables that were not significant in the multivariate analysis included gender, marital status, self-rated health, functional capacity, total social resources, number of informal helpers, feelings of loneliness, depressive symptoms, and stress rating.

TABLE 4. Logistic Regression Models Predicting Which Residents Are Worried About Relocation

Variable	Model 1		Model 2		Model 3	
	b	SE	b	SE	b	SE
Demographics						
Age	0.07***	0.02	0.07**	0.02	0.07**	0.03
Gender	0.30	0.36	0.33	0.39	0.39	0.42
Marital status	−0.54	0.37	−0.58	0.41	−0.37	0.44
Housing type	−1.25***	0.34	−1.14**	0.37	−1.14**	0.39
Financial security	0.63***	0.15	0.42*	0.17	0.41*	0.18
Physical health						
Self-rated health			−0.31	0.17	−0.12	0.19
Chronic conditions			0.15*	0.06	0.16**	0.07
ADL score			−0.02	0.20	0.03	0.20
IADL score			0.07	0.13	0.08	0.14
Psychological factors						
Social resources					−0.05	0.16
Informal helpers					−0.05	0.09
Loneliness					−0.23	0.28
Life satisfaction					−0.38*	0.25
Depression					0.06	0.08
Stress						
χ^2	52.66***		70.28***		82.22***	
−2LL	314.27		291.21		267.52	

Note. Gender, 1 = male, 2 = female. Marital status, 0 = not married, 1 = married. Housing type, 0 = apartment, 1 = other.
* $p < .05.$ ** $p < .01.$ *** $p < .001.$

DISCUSSION

In this study we report on interviews with older adults living in a suburban naturally occurring retirement community (NORC) who express concern regarding potential relocation from their current home. Over one quarter of the residents (26%) believe they may have to move over the next few years. The reasons they most commonly cite include failing health and financial constraints. Less common but still noteworthy are concerns about navigating safely around their residence, maintaining their home, and preserving social connections. The typical resident who is worried about relocation is an unmarried, older woman, living alone in an apartment rather than a home or congregrate housing, who feels insecure about her financial status. She has more chronic medical conditions, takes more prescription medications, and reports generally worse overall physical health. In addition, she is more functionally impaired, with a greater degree of dependency in both ADLs and IADLs. She has fewer informal caregivers available to provide assistance, a more constricted social network, and is less satisfied with life. Despite infrequent loneliness, she often feels depressed and describes her recent life experiences as stressful. Overall, then, we have a profile of residents worried about relocation who feel vulnerable on a number of fronts–financial, physical, social, and psychological. We do not know how many of these residents will actually move in the years ahead, but at this point it is clear that they feel at risk.

The proportion of residents worried about relocation in this sample is substantially higher than the 10% identified by Hunt and Ross (1990) in their study of an apartment-based NORC and the 2.3% reported by Colsher and Wallace (1990) in their study of rural Iowans. Differences in item wording might be responsible for the variability across studies. Colsher and Wallace, for instance, asked about definite plans to move, while our question was more hypothetical and focused on anxiety about moving. It may be that the residents in our neighborhood-based NORC feel particularly at risk for relocation due to a combination of their personal circumstances and the support services they perceive as available (or unavailable) in the community. In addition to the variables reported on here, we also documented service utilization in this sample and found no differences between worried and not worried residents, $t(318) = -.72, p = .47$, suggesting that worried residents are not receiving more formal assistance, despite their vulnerabilities. Perhaps available services do not match what residents think they need. Or perhaps the very limitations that make residents feel susceptible to relocation are obstacles to service utilization itself. On this point, additional qualitative research would be helpful.

The most common reason residents think they may have to move is a change in health status. That finding is consistent with retrospective research with older adults after they have moved (see for example, Brown et al., 2002; Gardner, 1994). In our sample, the concerns about physical health seem to refer mainly to physical impairments that may limit residents' ability to live independently and safely in their current home. The residents mention specific ailments, such as arthritis, circulatory problems, and urinary disorders that might one day interfere with independent functioning. Residents who currently have only mild forms of these conditions, but are aware of the possible long-term trajectory after observing friends or family cope with the same conditions, may recognize that future frailty may be impending. Residents also mention architectural barriers and liabilities in their homes, such as stairs that are difficult to navigate and the risk of falls in bath areas. The near majority of worried residents (49%) live in rental units, in which home modifications to accommodate greater physical frailty may be more complicated to accomplish given the reluctance of landlords to make modifications, residents' lack of knowledge regarding the Fair Housing Act of 1988, and fear of eviction on the part of older adults if they request changes. These multifaceted issues may contribute to the feeling of worry expressed by this group and warrant further study.

Also common are concerns about available financial resources. Residents in apartments are worried about increases in their rent, and those in condominiums fear fluctuation in their maintenance fee. Even residents who own their home are not immune to housing concerns: some residents are *overhoused*, living in large homes whose upkeep and maintenance are becoming too burdensome, particularly for people living alone. Unlike in other studies (see for example, Colsher & Wallace, 1990), annual income was not associated with worry about relocation. Yet residents who were worried about having to move did say they felt it was hard to make ends meet. An annual income figure may not predict anxiety about moving because even residents with high incomes may face eventual relocation. An older adult who has a relatively high annual income but also lives in an expensive house or apartment may be just as susceptible to relocation (albeit a different kind of relocation) than a resident with a low income in a less expensive living situation.

Residents who are worried about moving also appear more psychologically vulnerable, that is, more depressed and stressed. Interestingly, they seem to be less lonely than the other residents in the NORC, which may simply mean that their access to peers provides important affiliation, which they would lose if they moved. Moreover, that type of support is not likely to help them when it comes to relocation. After all, their friends are aging themselves, and while friends may provide beneficial emotional support, their ability to provide practical assistance is likely limited.

Implications

Although the worried residents in this sample differed *statistically* from the not worried residents on a number of characteristics, it is probably more useful to think of those differences as one of degree rather than kind. Even the worried residents we interviewed are not severely impaired at this point. They are beginning to see signs of changing health, but rather than acute medical illnesses, most report diffuse physical problems such as back pain and muscle aches that are beginning to limit their functional independence. Likewise, they are managing financially at the moment, but they wonder about the lengths to which they will be called upon to stretch their limited income in the future. In terms of social support, they have some contact with friends and family, but they recognize that a comprehensive support system is not in place should they need it. In this sense we may have captured a snapshot of residents on the verge of a shift in dependence.

The worried residents in this sample seem similar to the increasing number of older adults making anticipatory relocations, moves in preparation for an expected change in health or disability status (Choi, 1996; Krout, Moen, Oggins, & Bowen, 1998). This kind of move can be precipitated by an obvious and inevitable need for more services (e.g., in response to a diagnosis of a progressive dementia) but also might be prompted by a more vague sense of personal risk. The cumulative effect of minor life adjustments may, over time, signal to an older adult that his or her increasing vulnerability may one day necessitate relocation. Identifying older adults at risk for relocation *prior to the actual need* is critical if aging in place is to be achieved. Two initiatives are important in this regard: making services available and letting residents know about them (Gallagher & Truglio-Londrigan, 2004).

Rinehart (2002) argued that housing designed specifically for seniors can promote residents' satisfaction with their living environment *and* the use of support services. We would argue the same could be said of a larger living context such as an NORC neighborhood like the one studied here. An NORC may include a large number of older adults and a set of services available to them. Capitalizing on existing services–and perhaps developing new ones–may enable older adults to age in place. This will require social services that respond proactively, rather than reactively, to the needs of residents (Siebert, 2003). Social workers have an important role to play in making this happen, by identifying clients at risk for relocation and providing services that enhance their independence. Based on the concerns of the residents in this study, examples of services that could support aging in place in an NORC neighborhood include: home modification programs to promote functional independence in homes where residents already feel comfortable; activity and fitness programs that could be marketed to residents, not just as exercise per se but as a way to help them maintain their independence; financial counseling to help residents with budgeting, asset management, and taking advantage of financial assistance programs; psychological support via programs that enhance control and adaptive coping; and social support in the form of productive engagement in the community and meaningful connections with peers and family (when desired). Older adults overwhelmingly desire to age in place, and they are more likely to accept services if those services will enable them to remain independent (MacDonald, Remus, & Laing, 1994). While some of these services (and others, such as mental health counseling and transportation) were available to the residents we studied, these services tend to be underutilized. More client-centered research is needed to understand why services go unused, how clients perceive these services, and how better to market and maintain utilization.

Limitations

Despite the consistency of our findings with previous research, there are limitations associated with this study. First, this was a cross-sectional study, so it is not possible to untangle the direction of causality in our findings. For instance, we know that residents who think they may have to move in the next few years are less satisfied with their lives, but we cannot say whether that dissatisfaction preceded the expectation of relocation or followed it.

Second, the multivariate model we tested was, by necessity, limited due to the sample size. We included variables that previous studies have suggested are important, but missing are other variables that also might be predictive of relocation anxiety, such as more detailed assessments of available family assistance and formal service accessibility. It is also worth noting that among all of the variables we examined, only a small set was predictive of relocation anxiety in multivariate analyses. At a univariate level, many characteristics seem to distinguish residents who are worried about relocation from residents who are not worried. Those characteristics may be useful to practitioners who are trying to identify residents who need assistance. At a more theoretical level, broad constructs such as physical frailty or negative affect may be more useful for model building and hypothesis testing in this research area.

Third, there might have been conceptual overlap between our relocation question and other constructs, which could account for the associations between worry about relocation and depression, life satisfaction, and recent life stress. Perhaps the relocation question simply identified a group of worriers, with pessimistic things to say about most aspects of their lives. The only other variable at our disposal that might inform this possibility is self-rated overall stress, and on it ratings are indeed higher in the worried group compared to the not worried group ($M = 5.4$ versus 4.4, $t(322) = -3.43$, $p < .01$). Of course it may be that the causes of their stress are the very same factors that evoke worry about relocation (e.g., poor physical health, functional dependence, financial insecurity). With our cross-sectional data we are unable to pinpoint the direction of causality. Moreover, without ratings on dispositional traits such as neuroticism, we have no direct information about whether residents are "worriers" in general or worried just about moving.

A fourth limitation is that the characteristics of the sample may limit generalizability. Using data from the 2000 census, we were able to estimate that our sample is representative of the population of older adults in the larger neighborhood in terms of income (approximately 8% in our sample live below the poverty line, 7.7% in the corresponding census tract), race/ethnicity (95% in our sample are white, 95% in the neighborhood), and the proportion of residents with self-reported functional impairments (14.0% in our sample, 14.1% in the community). At the same time, our sample, compared to the larger community of older adults, includes older adults with more education (43.2% had a high school degree versus 29.3% in the community), current jobs (19.1% versus 15.6%), and more women (71% versus 59%), who are unmarried (66% versus 54%), and living alone (59.6% versus 33.4%). It is possible that our purposive sampling technique may have *underestimated* relocation anxiety given the relative health and wealth of our sample; or may have *overestimated* relocation anxiety by assembling a group of unmarried seniors living alone. It also is unclear whether the same predictors of relocation anxiety would emerge among residents in a different kind of NORC, such as an urban high-rise where resident characteristics as well as service options might differ. For instance, Hunt's (1988) report on an apartment-based NORC described a sample in which 80% of the older residents were widowed women living alone, a group whose relocation concerns might be different from those expressed by different kinds of residents living in a different kind of setting. Clearly, results from this study need to be replicated in other samples and locations.

Ideally, a study with more detailed assessments, a larger sample, and a longitudinal design that could follow residents prospectively, much like the one by Robison and Moen (2000), would provide valuable insight into predictors of relocation. Particularly useful would be follow-up with the current sample to track (a) whether residents have relocated, (b) what type of housing they relocated to, (c) what prompted their relocation, and, equally important, (d) whether it was the residents who were worrying about relocation who actually did move. This final point raises the topic of predictive utility. As social service providers and health care professionals try to identify who is at risk for relocation, it is worthwhile to ask what source (or sources) of information are most useful–objective assessments of functioning, informant reports from family members or paid care providers, or self evaluations from clients themselves? In the midst of trying to decide whether a resident *can* stay at home is the concomitant question of whether a resident *should* stay at home. Some relocation for some people can be beneficial, despite initial qualms. Even though older adults may be at first reluctant to move (and not all are), some relocations may result in improved access to services, a more manageable and satisfying living space, and greater proximity to friends and family, all enhancing well-being once the initial shock of the move subsides (Lawton, Brody, & Turner-Massey, 1978). Consistent with the philosophy of social work practice, a person-centered approach to the issue of relocation is needed.

In conclusion, with this study we have examined a group of older adults in the unique living environment of a neighborhood NORC. If even here, where older adults have congregated to be near services and supports and each other, residents still feel vulnerable to relocation, something is needed to address their felt vulnerability. Older adults prefer to remain in their own homes for reasons both practical and psychological, and effective social work practice involves responding to those reasons. Our research suggests that what may be needed are preemptive, community-based efforts to identify early the older adults at risk for relocation, rather than waiting for residents to access the formal service network after an event or crisis. Resident-focused programs may help empower older citizens to identify their own needs, seek services, and work with peers, family, and service providers to devise a plan to age in place.

REFERENCES

AARP. (2000). *Fixing to stay: A national survey on housing and home modification issues*. Washington, DC: Author.

Booth, A., & Amato, P. (1990). Divorce, residential change and stress. *Journal of Divorce & Remarriage, 18*, 205-213.

Brodman, K., Erdmann, A. J., & Wolf, H. G. (1960). *Cornell Medical Index manual*. New York: Cornell University Medical College.

Brown, J. W., Liang, J., Krause, N., Akiyama, H., Sugisawa, H., & Fukaya, T. (2002). Transitions in living arrangements among elders in Japan: Does health make a difference? *The Journals of Gerontology, 57*, S209-S220.

Callahan, J. J., & Lanspery, S. (1997). Density makes a difference: Can we tap the power of NORCs? *Perspective on Aging*, January-March, 13-20.

Chevan, A. (1995). Holding on and letting go: Residential mobility during widowhood. *Research on Aging, 17*, 278-302.

Choi, N. G. (1996). Older persons who move: Reasons and health consequences. *Journal of Applied Gerontology, 15*, 325-344.

Colsher, P. L., & Wallace, R. B. (1990). Health and social antecedents of relocation in rural elderly persons. *Journal of Gerontology, 45*, S32-S38.

Fillenbaum, G. G. (1988). *Multidimensional functional assessment of older adults: The Duke Older American Resource and Services Procedure*. Hillsdale, NJ: Erlbaum Associates.

Forbes, S. A., Hoffart, N., & Redford, L. J. (1997). Decision making by high functional status elders regarding nursing home placement. *Journal of Case Management, 6*, 166-173.

Gallagher, L. P., & Truglio-Londrigan, M. (2004). Community support: Older adults' perceptions. *Clinical Nursing Research, 13*, 3-23.

Gardner, I. L. (1994). Why people move to retirement villages: Home owners and non-home owners. *Australian Journal on Ageing, 13*, 36-40.

Glassman, M. H. (1998). Clinical issues in housing choice for vulnerable elders. *Journal of Geriatric Psychiatry, 31*, 37-54.

Greenbaum, L., Kahler, J., & Finkelstein, S. (2002). *Plainview-Old Bethpage Care Community-wide Survey*. New York: Jewish Association for Services for the Aged.

Groves, M. A., & Wilson, V. F. (1992). To move or not to move? Factors influencing the housing choice of elderly persons. *Journal of Housing for the Elderly, 10,* 33-45.

Hunt, M. E. (1988). Transition over time: Naturally occurring retirement community. In G. Gutman & N. Blackie (Eds.), *Housing the very old*. Burnaby, British Columbia: Gerontology Research Center, Simon Fraser University.

Hunt, M. E. (2001). Settings conducive to the provision of long-term care. *Journal of Architectural and Planning Research, 18,* 223-233.

Hunt, M. E., & Ross, L. E. (1990). Naturally occurring retirement communities: A multiattribute examination of desirability factors. *The Gerontologist, 30,* 667-674.

Johnson, R. A., Schwiebert, V. B., & Rosenmann, P. A. (1994). Factors influencing nursing home placement decisions: The older adults' perspective. *Clinical Nursing Research, 3,* 269-281.

Katzman, R., Brown, T., Fuld, P., Peck, A., Schechter, R., & Schimmel, H. (1983). Validation of a short orientation-memory-concentration test of cognitive impairment. *American Journal of Psychiatry, 140,* 734-739.

Krout, J. A., Moen, P., Oggins, J., & Bowen, N. (1998). Reasons for relocation to a continuing care retirement community. *Pathways Working Paper No. 2*. Ithaca: Bronfenbrenner Life Course Center, Cornell University.

Lawler, K. (2001). *Aging in place: Coordinating housing and health care provision for America's growing elderly population*. Boston, MA: Harvard Joint Center on Housing Studies and Neighborhood Reinvestment Corporation.

Lawton, M. P., Brody, E. M., & Turner-Massey, P. (1978). The relationships of environmental factors to changes in well-being. *The Gerontologist, 18,* 133-137.

Lesher, E. L., & Berryhill, J. S. (1994). Validation of the Geriatric Depression Scale-Short Form among inpatients. *Journal of Clinical Psychology, 50,* 256-260.

Litwak, E., & Longino, C. F. Jr. (1987). Migration patterns among the elderly: A developmental perspective. *The Gerontologist, 27,* 266-272.

Lutgendorf, S. K., Reimer, T. T., Harvey, J. H., Marks, G., Hong, S., Hillis, S. L. et al. (2001). Effects of housing relocation on immunocompetence and psychosocial functioning in older adults. *The Journals of Gerontology, 56,* M97-M105.

MacDonald, M., Remus, G., & Laing, G. (1994). The link between housing and health in the elderly. *Journal of Gerontological Nursing, 20,* 5-10.

Miller, E. A., & Weissert, W. G. (2000). Predicting elderly people's risk for nursing home placement, hospitalization, functional impairment, and mortality: A synthesis. *Medical Care Research and Review, 57,* 259-297.

O'Bryant, S. L., & Murray, C. I. (1987). "Attachment to home" and other factors related to widows' relocation decisions. *Journal of Housing for the Elderly, 4,* 53-72.

Rinehart, B. H. (2002). Senior housing: Pathway to service utilization. *Journal of Gerontological Social Work, 39,* 57-75.

Robison, J. T., & Moen, P. (2000). Future housing expectations in late midlife: The role of retirement, gender, and social integration. In K. Pillemer, P. Moen, E. Wethington, & N. Glasgow (Eds.), *Social integration in the second half of life* (pp. 158-189). Baltimore: The Johns Hopkins University Press.

Siebert, C. (2003). Aging in place: Implications for occupational therapy. *OT Practice*, *8*, CE1-CE8.

U.S. Census Bureau. (2000). *Census 2000*. Retrieved October 28, 2002, from *http:factfinder.census.gov*.

Wiseman, R. F. (1980). Why older people move: Theoretical issues. *Research on Aging, 2,* 141-154.

Wright, R. E. (1995). Logistic regression. In L. G. Grimm & P. R. Yarnold (Eds.), *Reading and understanding multivariate statistics* (pp. 217-244). Washington, DC: American Psychological Association.

doi:10.1300/J083v49n01_10

HOUSING OUTCOMES

An Observation
of Assisted Living Environments:
Space Use and Behavior

Sheryl Zimmerman, PhD
C. Madeline Mitchell, MURP
Cory K. Chen, MA
Leslie A. Morgan, PhD
Ann L. Gruber-Baldini, PhD
Philip D. Sloane, MD, MPH
J. Kevin Eckert, PhD
Jean Munn, MSW

This research was supported by grants from the National Institute on Aging (RO1 AG13871, RO1 AG13863, K02 AG00970). The authors thank the facilities, residents, and families participating in the Collaborative Studies of Long-Term Care (CS-LTC), as well as Ms. Verita Custis Buie (University of Maryland, Baltimore) and Dr. Joan F. Walsh (University of North Carolina, Chapel Hill) who provided expert project coordination. Gratitude also is extended for data collection overseen by Betty Concha and conducted by Mary Alice McGurrin, Christine Schmitt, Ida Altman, Joan Bassler, Susan Baxter, Shirley Carter, Betty Dorsey, Diane Eagle, Susan Fallen, David Fallen, Jo Magness, Connie Nunamaker, Ronald Nunamaker, and Barbara Smith (University of Maryland, Baltimore), and for data management performed by Jane Darter (University of North Carolina, Chapel Hill).

[Haworth co-indexing entry note]: "An Observation of Assisted Living Environments: Space Use and Behavior." Zimmerman, Sheryl et al. Co-published simultaneously in *Journal of Gerontological Social Work* (The Haworth Press, Inc.) Vol. 49, No. 3, 2007, pp. 185-203; and: *Housing for the Elderly: Policy and Practice Issues* (ed: Philip McCallion) The Haworth Press, Inc., 2007, pp. 185-203. Single or multiple copies of this article are available for a fee from The Haworth Document Delivery Service [1-800-HAWORTH, 9:00 a.m. - 5:00 p.m. (EST). E-mail address: docdelivery@ haworthpress.com].

SUMMARY. Assisted living facilities have become increasingly popular for older adults needing assistance. They are intended to enable privacy and provide support, but the extent to which they do so, and the degree to which these relate to residents' needs, are unknown. This observational study of 1,830 residents in 182 facilities indicates that, during the mid-afternoon, the majority of residents are awake (79%), and one-half (49%) are awake and in public spaces. Residents who are cognitively and functionally impaired are more likely to be in public spaces, but less likely to be engaged. Residents who are awake and alone in private spaces are less likely to be impaired, but more likely to have medical conditions. Thus, residents needing more oversight seem to be positioned to obtain that oversight. doi:10.1300/J083v49n03_11 *[Article copies available for a fee from The Haworth Document Delivery Service: 1-800-HAWORTH. E-mail address: <docdelivery@haworthpress.com> Website: <http://www.HaworthPress.com> © 2007 by The Haworth Press, Inc. All rights reserved.]*

KEYWORDS. Residential care, activities, engagement, affect, depression, agitation, Cornell Scale for Depression in Dementia, Cohen-Mansfield Agitation Inventory

INTRODUCTION AND BACKGROUND

The mandate of assisted living (AL) is to meet the apparently conflicting goals of enabling privacy while facilitating interaction and providing oversight to attend to resident needs (Assisted Living Quality Coalition, 1998). This mission is relevant for the care of the 800,000 to 1.2 million residents of more than 33,000 facilities across the United States (Golant, 2004). There are differences in the extent to which privacy and services are provided, however, with a recent report noting that 27% of facilities offer comparatively few services and little privacy, and only 11% provide a great deal of both (Hawes, Phillips, Rose, Holan, & Sherman, 2003). This difference is possible because AL is expressly intended to include a broad range of care settings, thereby offering choice to suit consumer preferences. Consequently, these facilities range in size from small, converted private homes to multi-level campuses with many hundreds of beds, in which accommodations range from private apartments to multiple residents sharing a room (Hawes, Morris, Phillips, More, Fries, & Nonemaker, 1995; Morgan, Eckert, & Lyon, 1995). Thus, there is significant variability in the organization of space and the provision of privacy in AL. Further, the residents and their needs are diverse. Depending on the facility type, 15-37% of residents have at least one functional impairment; 23-42% have moderate or more severe cognitive impairment; 13% are depressed; and while more than 90% of residents participate in at least one social activity per week, those who are cognitively or functionally impaired do so less often (Watson, Garrett, Sloane, Gruber-Baldini, & Zimmerman, 2003; Zimmerman, Gruber-Baldini et al., 2003; Zimmerman, Scott et al., 2003).

While variability in the structure and process of AL is desirable in its ability to enable consumer choice, it is important to consider the match between what the facility offers and what the resident needs. In this person-in-environment (PIE) approach, well-being results from congruence or fit between environmental and personal characteristics (French, Caplan, & Harrison, 1982; Parmelee & Lawton, 1990). For example, high privacy–although of unquestionable value as a basic human right–may limit opportunities for oversight and social engagement for an impaired resident. For these and other institutionalized residents, social interaction in the facility may be especially important, because contact with family members and friends decreases by as much as one-half following admission to a long-term care facility (Port et al., 2001).

The benefit of social interaction has long been recognized. Settings that encourage supportive interpersonal relationships are associated with better resident function, and social engagement is associated with multiple positive outcomes including decreased mortality, slowed functional decline, and less depression and agitation (Beck et al., 1998; Berkman & Syme, 1979; Blazer, 1982; Cohen-Mansfield, Marx, & Werner, 1992; Mitchell & Kemp, 2000; Noelker & Harel, 1978; Pruchno & Rose, 2000; Unger, Johnson, & Marks, 1997). Pursuing strategies to reduce aggression is especially helpful, as aggression can disrupt the residential environment, resulting in the use of physical and chemical restraints (Menon et al., 2001; Heeren et al., 2003). Further, the nature and degree of interaction between residents and staff, and among residents themselves, is a strong predictor of quality of life (Mitchell & Kemp, 2000). In fact, in the presence of strong social support, the effects of functional impairment and poor health on depression and life satisfaction are mitigated (Cummings, 2002).

Although there is some evidence that components of the environment are related to social interactions (Cutchin, Owen, & Chang, 2003), few studies have specifically attempted to relate space use or environmental characteristics to social or affective behaviors. Nonetheless, design professionals have long encouraged AL developers to use space to encourage social interaction (Regnier & Scott, 2001). Given the importance of this issue and the lack of information on this topic, this paper will describe the observed use of space and its association with resident social and affective behaviors in AL, and examine their relationship to facility and resident characteristics. Attention will be given to those residents who are awake and alone in private spaces, to consider whether their level of impairment is such that more opportunity for oversight may be indicated. Also, the validity of observations of affect and agitation as obtained through a brief walk-through will be addressed by comparisons of these data with validated reported measures of depression and agitation. Finally, the implications of these findings for research and social work practice will be addressed.

METHODS

Design and sample. Data for this study were collected by the Collaborative Studies of Long Term Care (CS-LTC), a program of AL research in four states (Florida [FL], Maryland [MD], New Jersey [NJ], and North Carolina [NC]). The CS-LTC defined AL as facilities or discrete portions of facilities, licensed by the state at a non-nursing home level of care, that provide room, board, 24-hour oversight, and assistance with activities of daily living. A multi-level sampling frame was used to select facilities and residents for participation. Within each state, a representative region was identified, and a sampling frame was constructed consisting of all licensed AL facilities within each region. Facilities were sampled in the following three strata to reflect the broad range of AL: (1) facilities with < 16 beds; (2) facilities with > 16 beds of the *new-model* type (i.e., meant to capture the type of facilities proliferating under the recent surge of AL, and having criteria identified in a pilot study that differentiate them from other facilities [having been built after 1/1/87 and having at least one of the following components: at least two different monthly private pay rates; 20% or more of the residents requiring assistance with transfer; 25% or more of the residents who are incontinent daily; and either a registered or licensed nurse on duty at all times]); and (3) *traditional* facilities with > 16 beds, not meeting new-model criteria.

The sample was constructed to study approximately equal numbers of residents from each facility type; as a result, more smaller facilities (n = 113) were enrolled compared with the other facility types (n = 40 traditional and 40 new-model facilities). Within the sampling frame, facilities were randomly selected for participation; the overall recruitment rate was 59%, and differences between participating and nonparticipating AL facilities were minimal (e.g., nonparticipating facilities housed a slightly less impaired resident population, such that 4.6% vs. 9.9% were chairfast and 1.2% vs. 4.2% were unable to transfer). There were no significant differences in reference to proprietary status; affiliation with other long-term care facilities; facility age, size, or occupancy rate; and resident age, ethnicity or race.

Residents were eligible for study if they were 65 years of age or older. In smaller facilities, all residents were asked to participate; in larger facilities, residents were randomly chosen to a maximum of 20 subjects. Consent was obtained from residents or a responsible party (for those residents who were cognitively impaired), and the overall participation rate was 92%. Baseline data of 2,078 residents were collected from October 1997 through November 1998. Further details about the CS-LTC sampling and data collection procedures are available elsewhere (Zimmerman et al., 2001).

Facility administrators and primary care providers were interviewed on-site to obtain information regarding facility characteristics (proprietary status; presence of a registered or licensed nurse [RN, LPN]; provision of social activities) and resident characteristics (age; co-morbid conditions; functional, cognitive, behavioral, affective status). Observations were conducted of the physical environment and resident location (*public vs. private space*), alertness (*awake vs. not*), social behaviors (*with others vs. alone* and *engaged vs. unengaged*), and affective behaviors (*negative affect vs. not* and *agitated vs. not*).

Facility characteristics. Administrators reported on the social and recreational activities provided by their facility using the *Availability of Social and Recreational Activities* scale of the Policy and Program Information Form (POLIF) (Moos & Lemke, 1994). The thirteen items included in this scale (exercise and physical fitness; outside entertainment; discussion groups; reality orientation groups; self-help groups; movies; club, drama, singing groups; classes or lectures; bingo, cards, other games; parties; religious services; social hour; arts and crafts were summed into an aggregate measure indicating the percentage of items that were available. If more than 25% of the items were missing, the measure was not calculated. For facilities missing some items, but fewer than 25% of items, a percentage of positively scored non-missing items was calculated.

Data related to environmental characteristics were gathered by observation using the Therapeutic Environment Screening Survey-Residential Care (TESS-RC). This measure is a refinement of a similar nursing home (NH) measure, the TESS-NH (Sloane et al., 2002), and is completed through a structured observation of the facility. The TESS-RC yields a summary score, the Assisted Living Environmental Quality Score (AL-EQS), a 15-item scale including items such as facility cleanliness, homelikeness, and privacy (alpha = .75). For both the TESS-RC and the AL-EQS, a dichotomous variable was created using the median scores, 18 and 6, respectively, to divide the facilities into two groups. In this study, the low scores were those that fell below the median score.

Resident characteristics. Care providers provided information on the presence/absence of 31 medical conditions, which were summarized as a single comorbidity index. They also reported on functional status with eight activities of daily living (ADL) items from the Minimum Data Set (MDS) that assess dependency over the last seven days: in bed mobility, eating, locomotion, transfer, toileting, dressing, personal hygiene and bathing (Morris, Fries, & Morris, 1999). In these analyses, "dependent" was computed as a dichotomous variable, indicating whether or not the resident needed limited or extensive assistance, or was totally dependent, on three or more ADLs. Also, a summary functional status score ranging from 0 to 8 was computed indicating the total number of ADLs in which the resident was dependent. (Here and for the variables below, dichotomized data are used for ease of interpretation and continuous data are used for purposes of adjustment.) Cognitive status was assessed with the Minimum Data Set Cognition Scale (MDS-COGS), and computed as a dichotomous variable using a cut-point of five to indicate severe impairment (Hartmaier, Sloane, Guess & Koch, 1994). Behavioral status was measured with the Cohen-Mansfield Agitation Inventory (CMAI), a scale that identifies the frequency of reported agitated behaviors (pacing, loud verbal excess, non-loud verbal excess, repetitive mannerisms, physical aggression, socially inappropriate behaviors, rummaging, and other negative behaviors) over the last two weeks (Cohen-Mansfield, 1986); a dichotomous agitation variable, indicating that at least one behavior had occurred, was created for these analyses. For adjustment purposes, a sum of the fourteen agitation items was used. Affective status was determined using the Cornell Scale for Depression in Dementia (CSD-D), a scale of depressive symptomatology designed to rate depression in persons with dementia; the CSD-D consists of 19 items, each scored 0-2, and dichotomized such that scores 8 or higher are considered to be indicative of depression (Alexopoulos, Abrams, Young, & Shamoian, 1988).

In addition, each resident's location, alertness, and social and affective behaviors were observed during a snap-shot walkthrough of the facility. A total of 1,830 residents in 182 facilities were observed for 10-20 seconds each, between 2:00 and 4:30 in the afternoon (when personal care and meals were not expected to occur). In total, 1,962 of the 2,078 residents (94%) in 192 facilities were actually observed; however, data from 132 residents are not included in these analyses because 81 were missing a time indicator and 51 were conducted outside of the prescribed 2:00-4:30 time window. Location was coded as *public vs. private space*, with public space including outdoor areas (although only 2% of the residents were outdoors). Alertness was coded as *awake vs. not*, the latter including residents who were either asleep (13%) or drowsy (8%) at the time of the observation. Social behaviors included *being alone vs. being with others* (i.e., in a room without others or in a room with others but further than ten feet away from others and not engaged in an activity with them, vs. other) and *being engaged vs. being unengaged* (i.e., active [43%], watching [27%], or involved in one-on-one care [1%] vs. being idle). One of the affective behaviors (*negative affect vs. not*) was coded based on the Philadelphia Geriatric Center Affect Rating Scale (Lawton, Van Haitsma, & Klapper,

1996), as negative (anxiety/fear [3%], sadness [2%], and anger [1%]), vs. positive (pleasure [10%], contentment [34%], interest [31%] and sleeping/dozing [19%]. The other affective behavior (*agitated vs. not*) was observed and coded based on the CMAI (Cohen-Mansfield, 1986), and dichotomized as either none or some agitated behaviors observed.

Analyses. Descriptive statistics were computed for each variable, overall and for those residents who were awake during the observation period. Bivariate relationships between facility characteristics and resident characteristics, and resident use of space, alertness and behavior, were examined using the chi-square statistic. To better understand the relationships between facility characteristics and resident behaviors, adjusted odds ratios were computed adjusting for resident functional status (ADL summary score); cognitive status (MDS-COGS); behavioral status (CMAI summary score); affective status (CSD-D); and age, gender, and comorbidity (comorbidity summary score). Bivariate comparisons between residents who were in private spaces, awake and alone versus all other awake residents were made using the chi-square statistic for categorical variables and the t-test for continuous variables. Odds ratios adjusted for resident characteristics were also computed for residents alone and awake in private spaces, for the facility characteristics under study. All analyses were conducted using software developed by the Statistical Analysis System (SAS; SAS Institute Inc., 1999), except for those calculating odds ratios, which used Stata to adjust for multiple resident observations within a facility (StataCorp., 2001).

RESULTS

Table 1 shows the distribution of facility and resident characteristics. The majority of facilities were for-profit (84%) and slightly less than one-half had an RN or an LPN on staff (47%). On a scale ranging from 0-26, their mean environmental quality score was 16.3 (SD 5.2), and administrators reported providing an average of 5.8 (SD 3.3) of 13 social and recreational activities. The residents in these analyses were overwhelming female (76%), averaged 84.0 (SD 7.7) years of age, and had an average of 4.6 (SD 2.7) comorbidities. Based on care provider report, 31% were dependent in at least one ADL; 24% were severely cognitively impaired; 42% were agitated, and 14% were depressed. The 1,830 residents who were observed did not differ from the larger cohort of 2,078 residents on any of these variables.

During the mid-afternoon, three-quarters (79%) of the residents were awake. These residents more often were in public spaces (63%), with others (59%),

TABLE 1. Characteristics of Assisted Living Facilities (N = 182) and Residents (N = 1,830) Participating in the Observational Component of the Collaborative Studies of Long-Term Care

	Number (%) or mean (SD)
Facility characteristics[a]	
Facility type, <16 beds	108 (59.3%)
Traditional	36 (19.8%)
New-model	38 (20.9%)
Administration, for profit	152 (84.0%)
Staffing, have RN/LPN	68 (46.6%)
Physical environment, ALEQS, mean (SD)	16.3 (5.2)
low, as per median split	100 (54.9%)
Social environment, activities, mean (SD)	5.8 (3.3)
low, as per median split	88 (48.9%)
Resident characteristics[a]	
Age	84.0 (7.7)
Female	1388 (76.1%)
Comorbidities, of 31 conditions	4.6 (2.7)
Functional status, MDS-ADL, number (%) dependent	552 (31.0%)
mean (SD)	2.0 (2.3)
Cognitive status, MDS-COGS, number (%) severely impaired	438 (24.4%)
mean (SD)	2.7 (2.9)
Behavioral status, CMAI, number (%) agitated	767 (42.2%)
mean (SD)	1.5 (2.5)
Affective status, CSD-D, number (%) depressed	252 (13.9%)
mean (SD)	3.3 (4.5)

[a] Number missing ranges from 0-36 (facility-level) and 1-32 (resident-level).

engaged (89%), and not displaying negative affect (93%) or agitation (94%) (see Table 2).

As shown on Table 3, residents were more often in public spaces and with others if they were in facilities that were smaller (69% compared to 50% in traditional and new-model facilities), for-profit (60% vs. 45%), did not have a nurse on staff (68% vs. 47%), and had poorer environmental quality (64% vs. 50%) (all p < .001). Reported provision of activities did not relate to the proportion of residents in public spaces or with others; however, in facilities with more activities, more residents were observed to be awake (84% vs. 72%) and engaged (92% vs. 84%), and fewer were agitated (3% vs. 9%) (all p < .001). Traditional facilities had the fewest residents who were engaged (85% vs. 88-92%) and agitated (4% vs. 5-9%) (both p < .01).

The residents' reported status was consistently related to observed use of space and behavior. Residents who were functionally impaired were more likely to be in public spaces (62% of dependent vs. 54% of independent individuals

TABLE 2. Space Use and Social and Affective Behaviors of Awake Residents

	Number	Percent
Awake residents (total observed = 1830)	1436	78.5%
Of residents who were awake (1436):		
Space use[a]		
Public space	900	62.9%
Private space	531	37.1%
Social behaviors[a]		
With others	850	59.3%
Alone	583	40.7%
Engaged	1276	88.9%
Unengaged	160	11.1%
Affective behaviors[a]		
Negative affect	99	7.0%
No negative affect	1334	93.0%
Agitated	84	5.9%
Not agitated	1352	94.2%

[a] Number missing ranges from 0-5.

were in public spaces, p < .001), as were those with cognitive and behavioral problems (69% vs. 52% and 63% vs. 51%, respectively). More highly impaired residents were also less likely to be awake (percents related to functional impairment, cognitive impairment, and depression range from 71-73%, vs. 79-82% for those not impaired; all results significant), and if awake, were more likely to be with others and displaying negative affect and agitation. The related figures are provided on Table 4.

Adjusted odds ratios (Table 5) indicate that, controlling for reported resident status, residents in public spaces were almost twice as likely to reside in facilities that were small as opposed to new-model (AOR = 1.9, p < .001) and 30% more likely to reside in facilities that report providing more social activities (p < .05). Also, they were more likely to be in a private space if the facility had an RN or LPN (p < .001) or a higher environmental score (p < .01). A higher environmental score also correlated to more residents being awake (AOR = 1.4, p < .01), as did the reported provision of more services (AOR = 1.5, p < .001). No facility characteristics correlated to observed affect or agitation, but residents in smaller and traditional facilities were approximately one-half as likely to be engaged as those in new-model facilities (p < .05); and those in facilities that provided more activities were more than twice as likely to be engaged (AOR = 2.3, p < .001). Finally, those in for-profit facilities were 60% more likely to be with others (p < .05).

Residents, who are in private spaces, awake and alone, merit special attention if their social, affective, or functional status suggests a need for oversight or involvement. Of those who were awake and alone in private spaces (Table 6),

TABLE 3. Resident Space Use, Alertness, and Behavior by Facility Characteristics (N = 1830)

Percent of residents:	Facility Type				Administration			Staffing			Physical Environment			Social Environment		
											ALEQS Median split			Activities Median split		
	<16 Beds (n = 614)	Traditional (n = 533)	New-Model (n = 683)	p	For-profit (n = 1383)	Not-for-profit (n = 440)	p	RN/LPN Yes (n = 987)	RN/LPN No (n = 499)	p	Low (n = 790)	High (n = 1040)	p	Low (n = 812)	High (n = 1011)	p
Location																
Public space	68.6%	49.8%	50.1%	***	59.6%	45.4%	***	47.3%	68.0%	***	64.0%	50.3%	***	56.0%	56.3%	
Alertness																
Awake	76.9%	79.0%	79.5%		77.4%	82.7%	*	79.2%	78.0%		75.3%	80.9%	**	72.2%	83.5%	***
Of residents who were awake (N = 1436):																
Social behaviors																
With others (n = 850)	65.6%	57.1%	55.5%	**	62.9%	48.5%	***	55.7%	64.5%	**	64.9%	55.4%	***	60.1%	58.7%	
Alone (n = 583)	34.4%	42.9%	44.5%		37.1%	51.5%		44.3%	35.5%		35.1%	44.6%		39.9%	41.3%	
Engaged (n = 1276)	88.4%	85.0%	92.3%	**	89.0%	88.7%		89.4%	88.2%		88.9%	88.8%		83.8%	92.3%	***
Unengaged (n = 160)	11.6%	15.0%	7.7%		11.0%	10.9%		10.6%	11.8%		11.1%	11.2%		16.2%	7.7%	
Affective behaviors																
Negative affect (n = 99)	6.8%	5.7%	7.9%	**	7.4%	5.5%		5.6%	8.0%		7.6%	6.4%		9.5%	5.1%	***
No negative affect (n = 1317)	93.2%	94.3%	92.1%		92.6%	94.5%		94.4%	92.0%		92.4%	93.6%		90.5%	94.9%	
Agitated (n = 84)	8.5%	3.6%	5.3%	**	6.4%	4.1%		5.0%	6.9%	.	7.2%	4.9%		9.4%	3.4%	***
Not agitated (n = 1352)	91.5%	96.4%	94.7%		93.6%	95.9%		95.0%	93.1%		92.8%	95.1%		90.6%	96.6%	

* p ≤ .05, ** p ≤ .01, ***p ≤ .001

TABLE 4. Resident Space Use, Alertness, and Behavior by Reported Resident Characteristics (N = 1830)

Percent of residents:	Functional Impairment (ADLs)			Cognitive Impairment (MDS-COGS)			Agitation (CMAI)			Depression (CSD-D)		
	Dependent (n = 552)	Not Dependent (n = 1225)	p	Severe (n = 438)	Not Severe (n = 1360)	p	Agitated (n = 767)	Not Agitated (n = 1051)	p	Depressed (n = 250)	Not Depressed (n = 1561)	p
Location												
Public space	62.3%	53.6%	***	68.9%	52.0%	***	63.4%	50.7%	***	60.0%	55.4%	
Alertness												
Awake	71.8%	81.9%	***	70.9%	81.3%	***	76.7%	79.8%		73.0%	79.4%	*
Of residents who were awake (N = 1436):												
Social behaviors												
With others (n = 827)	63.2%	57.2%	*	72.0%	55.2%	***	63.8%	55.9%	**	66.9%	58.0%	*
Alone (n = 574)	36.8%	42.8%		28.0%	44.9%		36.2%	44.1%		33.2%	42.0%	
Engaged (n = 1248)	84.9%	90.5%	**	84.7%	90.0%	**	88.3%	89.3%		84.8%	89.5%	
Unengaged (n = 156)	15.1%	9.5%		15.3%	10.0%		11.7%	10.7%		15.2%	10.5%	
Affective behaviors												
Negative affect (n = 94)	12.1%	4.6%	***	13.0%	4.9%	***	10.9%	3.9%	***	15.8%	5.5%	***
No negative affect (n = 1290)	87.9%	95.4%		87.0%	95.1%		89.1%	96.1%		84.2%	94.5%	
Agitated (n = 82)	13.6%	2.8%	***	16.6%	2.6%	***	9.9%	3.0%	***	9.8%	5.2%	*
Not agitated (n = 1322)	86.4%	97.2%		83.4%	97.4%		90.1%	97.0%		90.2%	94.8%	

* p ≤ .05, ** p ≤ .01, ***p ≤ .001

TABLE 5. Adjusted Odds Ratios of Resident Space Use, Alertness, and Behavior by Facility Characteristics (N = 1830)[a]

	Facility Type				Administration		Staffing		Physical Environment		Social Environment	
	< 16 beds vs. New-model		Traditional vs. New-Model		For-profit		Have RN/LPN		ALEQS Score (Median split high)		Activities Score (Median split high)	
	AOR	p	AOR	p	AOR	p	AOR	p	AOR	p	AOR	p
Location												
Public space vs. private (n = 1735)	1.9	***	1.0		1.5		0.5	***	0.7	**	1.3	*
Alertness												
Awake vs. not (n = 1752)	0.9		0.9		0.8		1.1		1.4	**	1.5	***
Of residents who were awake (N = 1436):												
Social behaviors												
With others vs. alone (n = 1381)	1.3		1.1		1.6	*	0.8		0.7		1.3	
Engaged (n = 1381)	0.5	*	0.4	*	1.0		1.3		1.1		2.3	***
Affective behaviors												
Negative affect (n = 1378)	0.6		0.8		1.0		0.8		1.0		1.0	
Agitated (n = 1381)	1.0		0.7		0.7		0.9		1.0		0.8	

[a] Adjusted for resident functional, cognitive, behavioral, and affective status; age; gender; and co-morbidity.
* $p \leq .05$, ** $p \leq .01$, *** $p \leq .001$

TABLE 6. Residents in Private Spaces, Awake and Alone, by Resident Characteristics (N = 1436)

	Private, Awake and Alone (n = 374)	All Awake Others (n = 1054)	
	Percent or Mean (SD)	Percent or Mean (SD)	p
Observed characteristic[a]			
Engaged	75.4%	93.6%	<.001
Unengaged	24.6%	6.4%	
Negative affect	8.6%	6.4%	.154
No negative affect	91.4%	93.6%	
Agitated	3.7%	6.6%	.041
Not agitated	96.3%	93.4%	
Reported characteristic[a]			
ADL dependent (MDS-ADL)	22.6%	30.4%	.004
Not ADL dependent	77.4%	69.6%	
Severe cognitive impairment (MDS-COGS)	12.2%	25.1%	<.001
Not severe cognitive impairment	87.8%	74.9%	
Agitated behavior (CMAI)	31.2%	44.6%	<.001
No agitated behavior	68.8%	55.4%	
Depressed (CSD-D)	11.0%	13.5%	.226
Not depressed	89.0%	86.5%	
Demographic characteristic[a]			
Male	22.3%	22.8%	.849
Female	77.7%	77.2%	
Age	84.8 (7.7)	83.3 (7.7)	.844
Co-morbid conditions	5.2 (3.0)	4.3 (2.6)	.001

[a] Number missing ranges from 8-40.

three quarters were engaged. Significantly fewer of those with severe cognitive impairment were awake and alone in private spaces (12% vs. 25% awake in public spaces and/or not alone; p < .001). More than 30% of those who were awake and alone in private spaces were reported to be agitated, but the proportion of residents reported to be agitated was higher for those in public spaces and/or not alone (45%; p < .001). A similar relationship was found for functional impairment (23% vs. 30%; p = .004), but not for comorbid conditions (mean 5.2 vs. 4.3; p = .001), and no relationship was evident for depression. Controlling for resident characteristics (Table 7), residents in smaller and for-profit facilities were less likely to be in private spaces, awake and alone (p = .052 and .015, respectively), whereas residents of facilities that had an RN or LPN and scored higher on the physical environment scale were more likely to be in private spaces, awake and alone (p = .001).

TABLE 7. Adjusted Odds Ratios of Residents in Private Spaces, Awake and Alone, by Facility Characteristic (N = 1436)[a]

	AOR	p
Facility type		
< 16 beds vs. New-model	0.7	.052
Traditional vs. New-model	0.9	.745
For-profit	0.6	.015
Have RN or LPN	2.1	.001
Physical Environment (high)	1.7	.001
Social Environment (high)	0.8	.134

[a] Adjusted for resident functional, cognitive, behavioral, and affective status; age; gender and co-morbidity.

DISCUSSION

During a snapshot observation of what was likely a typical afternoon in 182 AL facilities across four states, three quarters of all residents were awake and one-half of all residents were awake and in a public space. Slightly fewer were awake and with others (46%), but most (71%) were engaged (i.e., active, watching, or involved in one-on-one care). Being awake, in a public space, with others, and/or engaged are not inherently good or bad, except as they reflect resident choice and need–and outcomes, although these snapshot data do not lend themselves to such an analysis. This study did not assess resident choice, but it did assess potential need as reflected in reported levels of functional, cognitive, behavioral, and affective impairment.

A comprehensive PIE approach requires information and acknowledgement of personal preferences and values. In this approach, environmental characteristics determine the availability (supply) of resources, and personal values, desires, or goals determine the optimal use of these resources. In the simplest terms, a fit between supply and values is considered beneficial (produces higher levels of well-being), and a poor fit damages well-being, leading to stress and physical decline (French, Caplan, & Harrison, 1982). Ideally, the amount of privacy and opportunities for engagement (supply) provided within the AL environment (both social and physical) will be congruent with the resident's stated needs and values. In cases when cognitively impaired residents are not able to indicate their own personal preferences, staff must often rely upon observation of outcomes (e.g., agitation) to determine fit. If staff adjust the environment based on their observations, a recursive relationship between person and environment will occur. That is, personal values will shape the environment and the environment will shape the resident's personal experience.

For example, residents who are agitated in public (a poor outcome indicating poor PIE fit) may be moved into less stimulating (e.g., private) space.

Reported affective status did not relate to the use of space, but functional, cognitive, and behavioral status did–such that impaired residents were more likely to be in public spaces during the mid-afternoon. While this study can only speculate, it is plausible that facility practices and the environmental configuration of AL facilities are in part responsible for the increased use of public space by impaired residents observed in this study. Such positioning is advantageous, as public space affords staff oversight that private space does not. Thus, this finding suggests appropriate use of public vs. private space, as it might promote attention to more needy residents. Impaired residents also were more likely to be with others, but less likely to be awake and alert, and more likely to display negative affect and agitation. Taken together, these findings suggest facility staff have the opportunity (vis-à-vis location) to better engage impaired residents, and the cause to do so.

Another interesting finding is the relationship between facility characteristics and resident location, alertness, and social and affective behaviors. Residents were more often in public spaces and with others if they were in facilities that are smaller, for-profit, do not have a nurse on staff, and have poorer environmental quality. A likely explanation for these relationships is that they reflect the level of resident impairment, because smaller and for-profit facilities tend to house more impaired residents (Zimmerman et al., 2003a). The adjusted odds ratios, however, indicate that when resident status was controlled, persons residing in small (vs. new-model) facilities were almost twice as likely to be in public spaces, albeit 50% less likely to be engaged. In this regard, the restricted space of smaller facilities facilitates the congregation of residents in public areas; however, the space apparently is not being used to facilitate engagement. Other studies have found that residents of smaller facilities are more satisfied overall and more satisfied with social involvement than those in larger facilities, thereby highlighting the need to consider individual preferences as they relate to this matter (Chou, Boldy & Lee, 2003; Sikorska, 1999).

New-model facilities seem better able to facilitate engagement, and the manner in which they do so might provide guidance for other facility types. One such strategy is through service provision, which is higher (mean = 67%) than in smaller and traditional facilities (41% and 61%, respectively; Zimmerman et al., 2003a). Indeed, providing more activities was related to more use of public space, and more awake and alert residents, in adjusted analyses. These cross-sectional findings do not, however, establish whether the services that are provided reflect residents' proclivities (i.e., facilities that have more engaged residents will provide them more services) or whether the causal ordering is in the opposite direction (i.e., service provision itself increases engagement). The availability of activities has been related to resident engagement in other analyses, but the ordering of this relationship has not yet been established (Zimmerman et al., 2003b). A controlled trial could easily detect this relationship, and the findings might be used to improve the quality of AL care.

Considering that the majority of residents were in public spaces and that those with impairments were generally with others, what could be of particular concern is the status of those AL residents who are awake and alone in private spaces. This group, 20% of the entire sample, was less likely to be severely cognitive impaired, agitated, and functionally impaired, but more likely to have medical conditions. Thus, those residents needing more constant oversight (e.g., persons with dementia) seem to have been positioned to obtain that oversight. Further, controlling for resident characteristics and consistent with the finding related to medical conditions, those in facilities that had nurses were more often in private spaces, awake and alone when observed at the mid-afternoon. In sum, AL residents with more medical needs were either allowed to or sought privacy more than those with cognitive, behavioral, and/or functional needs.

An additional contribution of these analyses is as a validation of a brief walk-through observation. Residents reported to be agitated (on the CMAI) were more likely to be observed displaying agitated behaviors (10% vs. 3%; p = .001) and those reported to be depressed (on the CSD-D) were more likely to be displaying negative affect (16% vs. 6%; p = .001). Thus, the observational and report data serve as a test of concurrent validity, validating the ability of staff to report on these behaviors and of a brief walkthrough to be able to capture them.

There are limitations to the analyses reported here. The first is that the study did not evaluate how spaces were actually being used–for example, whether activities were occurring that might have related to or encouraged the use of public space. Also, the utility of the observational data notwithstanding, they are indeed but a snapshot. However, given how unlikely it is to capture infrequent events with such a snapshot, the findings most likely do reflect prevalent behavior, most indicative of how space is being used and how residents are behaving during the middle of an afternoon in AL.

Social workers are uniquely suited for advocating PIE fit in AL. Since Mary Richmond wrote *Social Diagnosis* (1917), social work as a profession has been identified with this theoretical perspective. Unfortunately, however, social workers are not visible in most AL settings, and while the National Association of Social Workers (NASW) was one of approximately 50 organizations comprising the recent Assisted Living Workgroup (ALW) appointed by the U.S. Senate, the workgroup's recommendations did not include the provision of social workers in these settings. Nonetheless, social workers are at times employed by, or consult with, AL facilities, and social work values are embedded in many of the core ALW recommendations (e.g., protecting resident rights; supporting dignity, autonomy, and independence; and providing social services) (Assisted Living Workgroup, 2003). Indeed, the AL philosophy of service delivery emphasizes the values of individual choice and quality of life, which are central to social work advocacy in other settings. The focus of this paper–the use of space to create an optimal social environment for residents–is a point for which social work advocacy, in the tradition of Mary Richmond, may serve the increasing numbers of AL residents well.

REFERENCES

Alexopoulos, G. S., Abrams, R. C., Young, R. C., & Shamoian, C. A. (1988). Cornell Scale for Depression in Dementia. *Biological Psychiatry, 23*(3), 271-284.

Assisted Living Quality Coalition. (1998). *Assisted living quality initiative. Building a structure that promotes quality.* Washington, DC: Public Policy Institute, American Association of Retired Persons.

Assisted Living Workgroup. (2003). *Assuring quality in assisted living: Guidelines for federal and state policy, state regulation, and operations. A report to the U.S. Senate Special Committee on Aging.* Washington, DC.

Beck, C., Frank, L., Chumbler, M. R., O'Sullivan, P., Vogelpohl, T. S., Rasin, J. et al. (1998). Correlates of disruptive behavior in severely cognitively impaired nursing home residents. *Gerontologist, 38*(2), 189-198.

Berkman, L. F., & Syme, S. L. (1979). Social networks, host resistance, and mortality: A nine year follow up study of Alameda County residents. *American Journal of Epidemiology, 109*(2), 186-204.

Blazer, D. G. (1982). Social support and mortality in an elderly community population. *American Journal of Epidemiology, 115*(5), 684-694.

Chou, S. C., Boldy, D. P., & Lee, A. H. (2003). Factors influencing residents' satisfaction in residential aged care. *Gerontologist, 43*(4), 459-472.

Cohen-Mansfield, J. (1986). Agitated behaviors in the elderly. II. Preliminary results in the cognitively deteriorated. *Journal of the American Geriatrics Society, 34*(10), 722-727.

Cohen-Mansfield, J., Marx, M. S., & Werner, P. (1992). Agitation in elderly persons. An integrative report of findings in a nursing home. *International Psychogeriatrics, 4*, 221-240.

Cummings, S. M. (2002). Predictors of psychological well-being among assisted-living residents. *Health and Social Work, 27*(4), 293-302.

Cutchin, M. P., Owen, S. V., & Chang, P. J. (2003). Becoming "at home" in assisted living residences: Exploring place integration processes. *Journal of Gerontology: Social Sciences, 58B*(4), S234-S243.

French, J. R. P., Jr., Caplan, R. D., & Harrison, R. V. (1982). *The mechanism of job stress and strain.* New York: Wiley.

Golant, S. M. (2004). Do impaired older persons with health care needs occupy U.S. assisted living facilities? An analysis of six national studies. *Journal of Gerontology Series B Psychological Sciences and Social Sciences, 59*(2), S68-79.

Hartmaier, S. L., Sloane, P. D., Guess, H. A., & Koch, G. G. (1994). The MDS Cognition Scale: A valid instrument for identifying and staging nursing home residents with dementia using the minimum data set. *Journal of the American Geriatrics Society, 42*(11), 1173-1179.

Hawes, C., Morris, J. N., Phillips, C. D., Mor, V., Fries, B. E., & Nonemaker, S. (1995). Reliability estimates for the Minimum Data Set for nursing home resident assessment and care screening (MDS). *Gerontologist, 35*(2), 172-178.

Hawes, C., Phillips, C. D., Rose, M., Holan, S., & Sherman, M. (2003). A national survey of assisted living facilities. *Gerontologist, 43*(6), 875-882.

Heeren, O., Borin, L., Raskin, A., Gruber-Baldini, A. L., Menon, A. S., Kaup, B. et al. (2003). Association of depression with agitation in elderly nursing home residents. *Journal of Geriatric Psychiatry and Neurology, 16*(1), 4-7.

Lawton, M. P., Van Haitsma, K., & Klapper, J. (1996). Observed affect in nursing home residents with Alzheimer's disease. *Journal of Gerontology: Social Sciences, 51*(1), P3-14.

Menon, A. S., Gruber-Baldini, A. L., Hebel, J. R., Kaup, B., Loreck, D., Zimmerman, S. I. et al. (2001). Relationship between aggressive behaviors and depression among nursing home residents with dementia. *International Journal of Geriatric Psychiatry, 16,* 139-146.

Mitchell, J. M., & Kemp, B. J. (2000). Quality of life in assisted living homes: A multidimensional analysis. *Journal of Gerontology: Psychological Sciences, 55B*(2), 117-127.

Moos, R. H., & Lemke, S. (1994). *Group residences for older adults: Physical features, policies, and social climate.* New York: Oxford University Press.

Morgan, L. A., Eckert, J. K., & Lyon, S. M. (Eds.). (1995). *Small board-and-care homes: Residential care in transition.* Baltimore and London: The Johns Hopkins University Press.

Morris, J. N., Fries, B. E., & Morris, S. A. (1999). Scaling ADLs within the MDS. *Journal of Gerontology, Series A: Biological Sciences and Medical Sciences, 54*(11), M546-553.

Noelker, L., & Harel, Z. (1978). Predictors of well-being and survival among institutionalized aged. *Gerontologist, 18*(6), 562-567.

Parmelee, P. A., & Lawton, M. P. (1990). The design of special environments for the aged. In J. E. Birren & K. W. Schaie (Eds.), *Handbook of the psychology of aging* (pp. 464-488). San Diego: Academic Press.

Port, C. L., Gruber-Baldini, A. L., Burton, L., Baumgarten, M., Hebel, J. R., Zimmerman, S. I. et al. (2001). Resident contact with family and friends following nursing home admission. *The Gerontologist, 41*(5), 589-596.

Pruchno, R. A., & Rose, M. S. (2000). The effects of long-term care environments on health outcomes. *The Gerontologist, 40*(4), 422-428.

Regnier, V. A., & Scott, A. C. (2001). Creating a therapeutic environment: Lessons from Northern European models. In Zimmerman, S. I., Sloane, P. D. & Eckert, J. K.

(Eds.), *Assisted living: Need, practices, policies in residential care for the elderly.* (pp. 53-77). Baltimore: Johns Hopkins University Press.

Richmond, M. (1917). *Social diagnosis.* New York: Russell Sage.

SAS Institute Inc. (1999). SAS/STAT User's Guide, Version 8. Cary, NC: SAS Institute.

Sikorska, E. (1999). Organizational determinants of resident satisfaction with assisted living. *The Gerontologist, 39*(4), 450-456.

Sloane, P. D., Mitchell, C. M., Weisman, G., Zimmerman, S., Foley, K. M., Lynn, M. et al. (2002). The Therapeutic Environment Screening Survey for Nursing Homes (TESS-NH): An observational instrument for assessing the physical environment of institutional settings for persons with dementia. *Journal of Gerontology: Social Sciences, 57*(2), S69-78.

StataCorp. (2001). Stata Statistical Software: Release 7.0. College Station, TX: Stata Corporation.

Unger, J. B., Johnson, C. A., & Marks, G. (1997). Functional decline in the elderly: Evidence for direct and stress-buffering protective effects of social interactions and physical activity. *Annals of Behavioral Medicine, 19*(2), 152-160.

Watson, L., Garrett, J. M., Sloane, P. D., Gruber-Baldini, A. L., & Zimmerman, S. (2003). Depression in assisted living: Results from a four-state study. *American Journal of Geriatric Psychiatry, 11*, 534-542.

Zimmerman, S., Gruber-Baldini, A. L., Sloane, P. D., Eckert, J. K., Hebel, J. R. Morgan, L. A. et al. (2003a). Assisted living and nursing homes: Apples and oranges? *The Gerontologist, 43*, 107-117.

Zimmerman, S., Scott, A. C., Park, N. S., Hall, S. A., Wetherby, M. M., Gruber-Baldini, A. L. et al. (2003b). Social engagement and its relationship to service provision in residential care/assisted living. *Social Work Research, 27*, 6-18.

Zimmerman, S., Sloane, P. D., Eckert, J. K., Buie, V. C., Walsh, J. F., Koch, G. G., & Hebel, J. R. (2001). An overview of the collaborative studies of long-term care. In S. Zimmerman, P. D. Sloane, & J. K. Eckert, J. K. (Eds.), *Assisted living: Needs, practices and policies in residential are for the elderly.* (pp. 117-143). Baltimore, MD: Johns Hopkins University Press.

doi:10.1300/J083v49n03_11

The Effect of Housing on Perceptions of Quality of Life of Older Adults Participating in a Medicaid Long-Term Care Demonstration Project

Nancy Kelley-Gillespie, PhD
O. William Farley, PhD

SUMMARY. As the nation struggles with the great increase in the numbers of older adults, many questions arise about how to provide housing and long-term care options that will ensure the quality of life of older adults. This study demonstrates that older adults and their families perceive quality of life more positively once moved from a nursing home to an assisted living facility using Medicaid funds. Results of this exploratory study are promising and suggest that having housing options available across the continuum of care with individualized case management offers older adults the hope for "quality living." doi:10.1300/J083v49n03_12 *[Article copies available for a fee from The Haworth Document Delivery Service: 1-800-HAWORTH. E-mail address: <docdelivery@haworthpress.com> Website: <http://www.HaworthPress.com> © 2007 by The Haworth Press, Inc. All rights reserved.]*

This research was funded by the Utah State Health Department and the W. D. Goodwill Family Foundation.

[Haworth co-indexing entry note]: "The Effect of Housing on Perceptions of Quality of Life of Older Adults Participating in a Medicaid Long-Term Care Demonstration Project." Kelley-Gillespie, Nancy, and O. William Farley. Co-published simultaneously in *Journal of Gerontological Social Work* (The Haworth Press, Inc.) Vol. 49, No. 3, 2007, pp. 205-228; and: *Housing for the Elderly: Policy and Practice Issues* (ed: Philip McCallion) The Haworth Press, Inc., 2007, pp. 205-228. Single or multiple copies of this article are available for a fee from The Haworth Document Delivery Service [1-800-HAWORTH, 9:00 a.m. - 5:00 p.m. (EST). E-mail address: docdelivery@haworthpress.com].

KEYWORDS. Quality of life, older adult, elderly, nursing home, assisted living facility, long-term care, Medicaid

INTRODUCTION

The United States is experiencing a dramatic increase in the proportion of older adults within the population. There is a growing need for less restrictive, community-based housing alternatives across the continuum of care levels for older adults in need of long-term care and housing arrangements, regardless of income levels. Funding for these alternative housing arrangements and support services is limited. Therefore, exploring funding options (whether public, private, or some combination of the two) that may be cost-effective, or even cost-neutral, and elicit higher levels of independence and quality of life are necessary.

The rapid rate of growth of the aging population in the United States is unprecedented (Brink, 1997). The proportion of the population who are over the age of 65 has increased more than three-fold since the turn of the 20th century. In 2000, almost thirteen percent of the population was aged 65 or older (U.S. Census Bureau, 2000). By 2050, the number of older adults is expected to double from 35 million to possibly more than 70 million, or more than 20% of the population (Hooyman & Kiyak, 1999; Ozawa, 1999; Wright, 1999). Utah is also experiencing dramatic population changes. Utah is one of eight states in the nation projected to experience a "doubling effect" by 2020, where the number of people aged 65 and older will increase from 165,000 in 1993 to more than 334,000 in 2020 (495,000 in 2025) (Wright, 1999).

As the number of older people increases, there will be an increase in the demand for both formal and informal provisions of long-term care and support and housing options. An array of living arrangements, care options, and services will be necessary to meet the needs of older adults. Offering choices across the continuum of care levels is reliant on ample resources and involves maximizing the quality of life of older people (Brink, 1997; Bury & Holme, 1990; Eng, Pedulla, Eleazer, McCann, & Fox, 1997; Kane, 2001). According to Farquhar (1994), measuring the quality of life of the elderly will be an "increasingly urgent and worthwhile task because of the growing pressure on health, social, and economic resources which this population group [will] generate [in the coming decades]" (p. 142). As choices of care expand that are cost neutral, more emphasis will be placed on the quality of life promoted by different long-term care settings and housing arrangements. Therefore, understanding what constitutes quality of life and how to measure it comprehensively from multiple perspectives, across settings, and over time is essential to the future of long-term care and support of older adults.

"AGING IN PLACE"

An older person's quality of life is profoundly impacted by where s/he lives and the quality of care s/he receives. Residing in the community is often the desired choice of older adults who prefer to "age in place" or live out the rest of their lives in the comfort of their own homes. It is generally considered preferable to nursing home or other institutional settings because of individualized attention and presumed better quality of care. In addition, the older adults tend to desire residing in the community because of the familiarity and history of the environment, the belief that their independence and privacy will be maximized, and the belief that their contributions to the community will be continued (Barusch, 1991; Hughes & Guihan, 1990; Kane, 2001; Lucksinger, 1994; Rabiner, Arcury, Howard, & Copeland, 1997). Kane (2001) recognized that older people prefer to avoid typical nursing homes; family members experience guilt and anguish when they see no other choice but nursing home placement for their loved one because of the constraining circumstances of the nursing home, particularly the lack of privacy (e.g., shared rooms and baths) and the rigidity of routines of daily life. She also asserted that these constraints lead to learned helplessness that destroys the human spirit and creates listlessness, depression, and abandonment of efforts to exert control. Promoting the idea of keeping people at home or in the community rather than in a nursing home or institution, despite disability or finances, is based on the values of promoting the integrity, respect, dignity, and worth of a person (George, 1998; Kane & Kane, 2001; National Association of Social Workers, 1996). These values represent the quality or state of being worthy, honored, or esteemed and are consistent with optimizing the quality of life of the elderly (George, 1998).

The preference of older adults to reside in the community often contrasts with general practice; there seems to be a bias toward institutionalization, regardless of the inappropriateness of the placement (Barusch, 1991; Brink, 1997; Kane, 2001; Kane & Kane, 2001; Rabiner et al., 1997). For older individuals who have limited resources (e.g., low-income, little family support), this "drift" toward institutionalization is especially apparent. Traditionally, Medicaid has been the primary source of payment for long-term care of the low-income, frail elderly population. These payments have been strictly confined to care provided in institutional settings (e.g., nursing homes, transitional care centers, hospitals). The choice for this group of older adults to reside in the community is generally restricted and impacts their quality of life (Barusch, 1991; Brink, 1997; Kane, 2001; Kane & Kane, 2001; Rabiner et al., 1997).

Costs across the continuum of care levels for older adults are dramatically increasing. Although 80-90% of long-term care assistance is provided on an unpaid basis by family members and friends, public expenditures for long-term care have increased steadily over the past few decades. The United States does not have sufficient funding in place in either the public or private sectors to help older adults anticipate and pay for necessary long-term care services. As the need for and use of long-term care services further escalates during this century, new funding streams will need to be developed to help older adults and their families cope with the costs of long-term care. Looking at costs, care levels, and payment options is important to consider if quality of life is to be satisfactorily addressed by the aging service delivery system (Kane, 2001; Kane & Kane, 2001; Rabiner et al., 1997).

In order to maximize quality of life, quality of life needs to be understood and measurable. How is quality of life defined? What factors, including housing arrangements, impact the perceptions of quality of life of older adults? Knowing what constitutes quality of life for older adults will allow it to be measured in a more useful way and may seriously affect social policies and service delivery models pertaining to this population.

DEFINITIONS OF QUALITY OF LIFE

Assessing the quality of life in older people is challenging because as people age they become more differentiated, rather than alike (Franks, 1996). This makes finding common components that jointly contribute to a higher quality of life among older people a difficult task for researchers. Franks (1996) stated, "Quality of life is a variable that researchers refer to with great frequency, define with considerably different terminology, and measure with great difficulty" (p. 21).

Arnold (1991) found that quality of life definitions should consider the following attributes: physical functioning and symptoms; emotional functioning and behavioral dysfunction; intellectual and cognitive functioning; social functioning and the existence of a supportive network; life satisfaction; health perceptions; economic status; ability to pursue interests and recreation; sexual functioning; and energy and vitality. In addition, health status was also found to be a key component of quality of life.

Kane (2001) identified 11 domains for measuring quality of life: sense of safety, security and order, physical comfort, enjoyment, meaningful activity, relationships, functional competence, dignity, privacy, individuality, autonomy/choice, and spiritual well-being. Each outcome can be successfully measured in a positive or negative form. She added that "accentuating the positive is worthwhile; it is sadly narrow to define quality as the absence of negative outcomes" (p. 297).

Several factors associated with quality of life of older people have also been identified by Atchley (1991). They include: freedom of choice, maximum control over one's life, and involvement in decision making; recognition of individuality; right to privacy and fostering of human dignity; continuity with the past and continuation of normal social roles; stimulating environment; age-appropriate opportunities and activities; sense of connectedness between home, neighborhood, and community; and opportunities for enjoyment, fun, humor, and creativity.

Many authors have claimed that quality of life is best represented by health-related characteristics. Schipper, Clinch, and Powell (1990), cited in Rosenberg and Holden (1997), suggested that quality of life is characterized by:

> the functional effect of an illness and its consequent therapy upon a patient, as perceived by the patient. Four broad domains contribute to the overall effect: physical and occupational function, psychological state, social interaction, and somatic sensation. This definition is based on the premise that the goal of medicine is to make the morbidity and mortality of a particular disease disappear. We seek to take away the disease and its consequences, and leave the patient as if untouched by the illness. (p. 13)

> Health is commonly considered one of the most important determinants of overall life quality. (Bond, 1999; Cairl, Schonfeld, Becker, & Oakley, 1999; Kane & Kane, 2001; McDowell & Newell, 1987; Rosenberg & Holden, 1997)

As seen with these definitions, quality of life is a fluid concept and has several interpretations. There is a great amount of interrelatedness among these definitions of quality of life. For example, a person who suffers from a stroke (physical condition) may be limited in socializing or communicating with others (social status). Or, disabilities brought on by the stroke (physical condition) may lead to a state of depression or may impact on the person's self-concept (psychological well-being). Thus, the factors associated with the definitions of quality of life are often interconnected.

ENVIRONMENTAL PRESS AS A THEORETICAL FRAMEWORK

The concept of quality of life of older people can be viewed holistically within an environmental press framework. Environmental press, first introduced by Lawton and Nahemow in 1973, refers to the demands that social and physical environments make on the individual to adapt, respond, or change. It pertains to the fit between an individual and his or her social environment (Hooyman & Kiyak, 1999; Kane, 2001). Environmental press includes the notion of "competence" or level of mastery, which assumes that the interaction between the environment and an individual is mediated by the individual's capacity to function in areas of biological health, sensation-perception, motives, behavior, and cognition. To the extent that a person can reduce or increase the level of environmental press, adaptation occurs, and the individual maintains his or her level of well-being and quality of life (Hooyman & Kiyak, 1999; Kane, 2001).

Environmental press can be applied to diverse settings where older people interact and can range from low to high. For example, an institutional setting (e.g., nursing home), where a person is reliant on others for self-care and has few opportunities to stimulate the senses or challenge the mind, elicits very little environmental press (Hooyman & Kiyak, 1999). Other environments may create a higher level of environmental press such as an assisted living facility where one's degree of independence and self-structure continues to be fostered. In order to maintain one's sense of "competence" as described above, an older person needs to change as the demands of the environment change. Hooyman and Kiyak (1999) explained that,

> [i]ndividuals perform at their maximum level when the environmental press slightly exceeds the level at which they adapt. In other words, the environment challenges them to test their limits but does not overwhelm them. If the level of environmental demand becomes too high, the individual experiences excessive stress or overload. When the environmental press is far below the individual's adaptation level, sensory deprivation, boredom, learned helplessness, and dependence on others may result. (p. 7)

In either case, if too much or too little environmental press exists, the person or the environment must change if the individual's adaptive capacity is to be restored and quality of life enhanced.

An individual experiences optimal well-being when there is a balance between his or her needs and the characteristics of the environment and the environment's ability to meet those needs (Hooyman & Kiyak, 1999; Kane, 2001). This concept of a person-environment fit links individual well-being and quality of life to the degree of congruence between an older person's needs and the environment's ability to meet those needs (Braun & Rose, 1989). Difficulties exist in measuring this "fit" between person and environment. It is challenging yet imperative to consider multiple personal, environmental, and outcome items in determining quality of life of older adults with a scale that is meaningful across items and settings that also controls for both individual and environmental factors (Braun & Rose, 1989).

OVERVIEW OF FLEXCARE:
A MEDICAID LONG-TERM CARE DEMONSTRATION PROJECT

One program designed to provide optional and more flexible housing arrangements in the state of Utah is called FlexCare. The FlexCare program provides a less-restrictive, community-based housing alternative to nursing homes for older adults. Long-term care and support services are provided in the community to older adults who are eligible for Medicaid and nursing home placement. These care and support services are paid for out of Medicaid monies that have traditionally only been used to pay for the long-term care needs of older adults in an institutional setting, not for the same level of care to be provided to individuals in a community-based setting (e.g., own home, assisted living facility, sheltered care, group home, shared housing, boarder home, foster care).

FlexCare is designed to enable older adults to reside in the community with appropriate care services in place. The primary goal of the FlexCare program is to situate people in their own homes or family homes, assisted living facilities, or other community placements that are less restrictive than a nursing home or institutional setting. In so doing, FlexCare strives to promote and enhance the quality of life of long-term care recipients and to optimize their independence and choices. A more flexible use of Medicaid monies that pays for caregiving as well as other ongoing support services (e.g., home health care, respite care, adult day care, rehabilitative therapy, visiting nursing, mental health care) gives individuals an accessible resource to help them stay in the community.

PURPOSE OF STUDY

The purpose of the FlexCare program evaluation was to attempt to determine the level of quality of life of the individuals who were receiving FlexCare services and had transitioned to a non-institutional housing arrangement. In order to get a complete picture of the quality of life of the FlexCare program participants, the perspectives of the program participants and their designated family members/friends were studied. If the quality of life of program participants improved with individualized case management and a more community-based living arrangement such as an assisted living facility, it may then be viewed as a worthwhile program and one to be expanded so that other older adults have access to FlexCare services across the continuum of long-term care levels. Only FlexCare program participants who chose assisted living facility placements were included in the program evaluation.

RESEARCH QUESTIONS

In order to gain a better understanding of what quality of life means for older adults across the continuum of long-term care, the following research questions were addressed: (1) Do quality of life perceptions of older people utilizing Medicaid funds change when they are offered individualized care in a community-based housing arrangement as opposed to standardized nursing home care? (2) What factors are important to determining an older person's perception of quality of life?

METHODOLOGY

This pre/post study was exploratory in nature. It focused on the perceptions of quality of life of older adults from the perspectives of two target groups–older adults themselves and their designated family members/friends. These individuals were initially interviewed and surveyed between March and November, 2001. Follow-up interviews of participants and surveys of family members/friends and care providers were completed between July, 2001 and April, 2002.

Sample

The sample included 42 individuals accepted into the FlexCare program between the months of March, 2001 and November, 2001 and their 31 family members/friends who completed the questionnaires at both time periods. The method of selection used for this study was a nonrandom purposive sampling procedure. Individuals were recruited for the program evaluation at the time of enrolment into FlexCare as it was just starting its demonstration phase. The sample came from the first cohort of participants who entered the program. Participants were Medicaid-eligible and qualified for nursing home placement as determined by the Utah State Health Department. All had lived in an institutional setting for at least 30 days prior to enrollment in the FlexCare program. All individuals were residing either in Salt Lake or Davis counties in Utah. At baseline, participants were living in a nursing home. They were assessed for the FlexCare program with acceptance pending medical and financial eligibility. They had not yet been placed in a community-alternative living arrangement (i.e., assisted living facility) nor had they been provided supportive services via the FlexCare program. At follow-up, participants had been accepted into the FlexCare program, had moved to an assisted living facility, and had been receiving FlexCare services for approximately four months.

Data Collection Procedures

A personal interview approach was used to administer the questionnaires to FlexCare participants at baseline, prior to receiving FlexCare services, and again approximately four months after baseline when FlexCare services had been implemented. When possible, a designated family member/friend who was actively involved in the participant's life and showed the most interest in the welfare of the participant was chosen by the participant and the FlexCare case manager/nurse to participate in this study. Family members/friends completed the self-administered questionnaires mailed to them at baseline and follow-up.

Instrument

The Assisted Living Facility-Quality of Life/Quality of Care Index (ALF-QoL/QoC), developed in 1997, was used for this study. The ALF-QoL/QoC is a variation of the Wisconsin Quality of Life Index (W-QoLI) that was developed in 1993 (Becker, 1995; Becker, 1998; Becker et al., 1993; Becker, Shaw, & Reib, 1995; Diamond & Becker, 1999; Diaz & Mercier, 1996; Diaz, Mercier, Hachey, Caron, & Boyer, 1999). Building on the multidimensional character of the W-QoLI, the ALF-QoL/QoC was designed more specifically for use with older adults and is more versatile. According to the instrument's developers, it is designed to be used in any residential setting across the continuum of care levels, despite its name (personal telephone conversion with Dr. Marion Becker, principal investigator/instrument developer, July, 2000). The ALF-QoL/QoC questionnaire is a multifaceted measurement tool. It consists of multiple subquestionnaires of which the participant questionnaire and family member/friend questionnaire were used for this study. The general areas of quality of life addressed in this measurement instrument are: physical health, functional status, emotional well-being/life satisfaction, environmental characteristics, care and assistance, and facility/program service satisfaction. The instrument was constructed using sources of measurement from other established, validated assessment tools that are in the public domain, such as the SF-36 Health Survey (Ware & Sherbourne, 1992), GATES (Geriatric Assessment Testing and Evaluation System) (Cairl, Pfeiffer, & Keller, 1984), MDS (Minimum Data Set Version 2.0) (Brown, 1995), Life Satisfaction Scale (Neugarten, Havighurst, & Tobin, 1961), Geriatric Depression Scale (Brink, Yesavage, & Lum, 1982), Spitzer's Prime MD (Spitzer, Williams, Kroenke, Linzer, Verloin, Hahn, & Brody, 1995), and the Affect Balance Scale (Bradburn, 1969). The ALF-QoL/QoC is comprehensive, consisting of approximately 130 questions (of which 105 were actually included in the data analyses for this study) related to multiple dimensions of quality as well as multiple perspectives on quality of life. It was designed to expand the focus of quality of life assessments beyond one model (e.g., medical or psychosocial) and to blend multiple approaches to quality of life assessments (Cairl et al., 1999).

Data Analysis

Data from the interviews and mailed surveys were coded and entered into a data file. Each survey question was scored either as a dichotomous variable or as an interval level variable. Data were analyzed using the statistical software package SPSS (Statistical Package for the Social Sciences) (SPSS, Inc., 2003). Descriptive frequencies were calculated to show mean ratings for the various factors within each life domain category that may determine quality of life perceptions. Data were analyzed using paired samples statistical t-tests to determine which factors were associated with higher quality of life ratings from participants and family members/friends. Data were compared across target groups and settings over time. As such, responses of participants and family members/friends were compared over time (baseline and follow-up) and setting (nursing home and assisted living). Raw mean scores from the baseline (nursing home setting) and follow-up (assisted living setting) interviews were reported, along with the number of participants, changes in mean scores between baseline and follow-up, and score meanings. Mean score changes were considered significant at the $p < .05$ level.

RESULTS

Participants

The sample consisted of 14 males (33%) and 28 females (67%). The mean age of the group was 72.9 years with an age range from 43-101 (all but eight were 60 or older). Eighty-eight percent (37) of the sample was White. More than 90% (38) of the sample reported completing a maximum of some post-high school education. The majority (32, or 76.2%) of the sample claimed to be either divorced or widowed. The mean nursing home stay was 11.79 months with a reported range from 1-120 months. The mean number of previous long-term care placements prior to the latest assisted living residence for this study was 1.94 with a reported range of 1-7 placements.

Table 1 presents domains from the ALF-QoL/QoC questionnaire along with participants' baseline and follow-up raw mean scores, range of scores, mean change, significance, and meaning. Domains were created from several independent questions. Quality of life domains that were found to exhibit a statistically

TABLE 1. Quality of Life Domains–Participants' Raw Mean Scores in a Nursing Home and Assisted Living Facility, Range, Change, Significance, and Meaning (N = 42)

Domain	Mean Scores		Range	Change	Meaning
	Nursing Home	Assisted Living Facility			
Physical health	23.19	23.17	7-35	-0.02	Higher = Better health
Importance of environment	6.24	6.74	0-7	0.50*	Higher = Important
Importance of staff, care, and assistance	11.43	11.57	0-12	0.14	Higher = Important
Importance of activities and social relations	7.60	7.86	0-9	0.26	Higher = Important
Importance of choices	2.81	2.93	0-3	0.12	Higher = Important
Satisfaction with the environment	26.07	31.55	7-35	5.48*	Higher = More satisfaction
Satisfaction with staff and care	45.05	52.19	12-60	7.14*	Higher = More satisfaction
Satisfaction with activities and social relations	33.88	36.19	9-45	2.31*	Higher = More satisfaction
Satisfaction with choice	12.05	13.07	3-15	1.02*	Higher = More satisfaction
Satisfaction with facility	9.90	13.21	3-15	3.31*	Higher = More satisfaction
Emotional well-being (depression/anxiety)	2.29	1.79	0-5	-0.50*	Higher = More depressed
Quality of life/Life satisfaction	22.38	21.90	4-31	-0.48	Higher = More satisfaction
Functional status	33.36	33.05	0-44	-0.31	Lower = More independent
Psych medications	7.64	7.79	2-11	-0.14	Higher = Medications working better

*Changes in mean raw scores were significant at the p ≤ .05 level.

significant change between the baseline and follow-up scores included: *importance of the environment* ($t = -3.26$, p < .002), *satisfaction with the environment* ($t = -6.70$, p < .001), *satisfaction with staff and care* ($t = -5.52$, p < .001), *satisfaction with activities and social relations* ($t = -2.26$, p < .029), *satisfaction with choice* ($t = -2.47$, p < .018), *satisfaction with the facility* ($t = -8.11$, p < .001), and *emotional well-being* ($t = 2.34$, p < .024).

In addition to the *domain* factors listed in Table 1, several *single-item* factors were identified in the study as quality of life indicators. As can be seen in Table 2, ratings by the participants of virtually every single-item factor increased to "very important" at follow-up. The single-item factor of *ability to care for self* decreased its rating of "very important" from 88.1% at baseline to 83.3% at follow-up; *ability to make own decisions* decreased its rating of "very important" from 85.7% at baseline to 78.6% at follow-up. The single-item factor of *being treated as a person* maintained its rating of "very important" in determining quality of life perceptions at baseline and follow-up (71.4%). The single-item factor rated lowest at baseline and follow-up was *money*.

Family Members/Friends

The sample consisted of 31 family members/friends of the FlexCare participants who completed and returned their mailed questionnaires at the beginning of the study and again four months later; this reflects a 74% return rate. There were 23 (74%) females and 8 (26%) males in the sample. Twenty-four (80%) had attended some college with six (20%) having completed undergraduate or post-graduate degrees. As is typical for the state of Utah, 28 (93%) were White. Twenty-three (79%) were married and five (17%) were divorced or widowed. The age range of the family members/friends sample was 30-77, with the mean age being 55.31 years.

The family members/friends reported that 23 (74%) participants had lived in one facility prior to joining the FlexCare program. Five (16.7%) had lived in 2-4 facilities, while three did not answer this question. Twenty (65%) of the family members/friends indicated that the participant was completely involved in the decision to move to the assisted living setting. Another nine (20%) were somewhat involved, and only two family members/friends reported that the participant was not involved in the decision.

Table 3 shows the raw mean scores of family members/friends on each quality of life domain at baseline and follow-up, ranges of scores, mean changes, significance, and meanings. The domains of *importance of environment*, *staff activities*, and *choice* remained essentially level from baseline to follow-up. As with the participants, family members/friends scored several domains as

TABLE 2. Importance of Single-Item Factors in Determining Quality of Life as Reported by Participants: Nursing Home vs. Assisted Living Facility (N = 42)

Factors in Determining Quality of Life	Not at all Important				Slightly Important				Moderately Important				Very Important			
	Nursing Home		Assisted Living Facility		Nursing Home		Assisted Living Facility		Nursing Home		Assisted Living Facility		Nursing Home		Assisted Living Facility	
	#	%	#	%	#	%	#	%	#	%	#	%	#	%	#	%
Physical health	1	2.4	0	0	4	9.5	1	2.4	12	28.6	6	14.3	25	54.5	35	83.3
Mental health	0	0	0	0	2	4.8	1	2.4	10	23.8	9	21.4	30	71.4	32	76.2
Family/friends	0	0	0	0	2	4.8	3	7.1	11	26.2	7	16.7	29	69.0	32	76.2
Ability to care for self	0	0	0	0	1	2.4	1	2.4	4	9.5	6	14.3	37	88.1	35	83.3
Feelings about self	0	0	0	0	4	9.5	4	9.5	11	26.2	4	9.5	27	64.3	34	81.0
Being treated as a person	0	0	1	2.4	4	9.5	3	7.1	8	19.0	8	19.0	30	71.4	30	71.4
Ability to make own decisions/choices	1	2.4	0	0	2	4.8	1	2.4	3	7.1	8	19.0	36	85.7	33	78.6
Money*	1	2.4	2	4.8	5	11.9	3	7.1	15	35.7	12	28.6	19	45.2	25	59.5

* 2 participants did not respond to this item at baseline.

TABLE 3. Quality of Life Domains—Family Members/Friends Raw Mean Scores in a Nursing Home and Assisted Living Facility, Range, Change, Significance, and Meaning (N = 31)

Domain	Mean Scores		Range	Change	Meaning
	Nursing Home	Assisted Living Facility			
Importance of environment	6.65	6.81	0-7	0.16	Higher = Important
Importance of staff, care, and assistance	11.52	11.45	0-12	-.07	Higher = Important
Importance of activities and social relations	8.10	8.19	0-9	0.09	Higher = Important
Importance of choices	2.87	2.77	0-3	-0.10	Higher = Important
Satisfaction with the environment	28.77	32.90	7-30	4.13*	Higher = More satisfaction
Satisfaction with staff and care	49.41	52.97	12-40	3.56*	Higher = More satisfaction
Satisfaction with activities and social relations	31.83	36.77	9-45	4.94*	Higher = More satisfaction
Satisfaction with choice	11.50	13.43	3-5	1.93*	Higher = More satisfaction
Satisfaction with facility	12.07	14.28	3-15	2.21*	Higher = More satisfaction
Emotional well-being (depression/anxiety)	1.60	1.80	0-5	0.2	Higher = More depressed
Quality of life/Life satisfaction	19.68	18.45	4-31	-1.23	Higher = More satisfaction
Functional status	28.77	29.19	0-44	0.42	Lower = More independent

* Changes in mean raw scores were significant at the $p \leq .05$ level.

being significantly higher after participants joined the FlexCare program and were moved to an assisted living facility. Family members/ friends indicated improved ratings for *satisfaction with the environment* ($t = 4.2$, $p < .001$), *satisfaction with staff and care* ($t = 2.5$, $p < .018$), *satisfaction with activities and social relations* ($t = 2.45$, $p < .02$), and *satisfaction with the facility* ($t = 3.59$, $p < .001$). In addition to being more satisfied with the participants' living arrangements, the family members/friends indicated they were more satisfied with the *choices* they were able to make ($t = 3.16$, $p < .004$).

In addition to the *domain* factors, the family members/friends rated several important *single-item* factors that seemed to influence the participants' quality of life at baseline and follow-up. As can be seen in Table 4, the family members/friends increased or maintained their ratings of "very important" from baseline to follow-up on the following single-item factors: *family/friends, ability to care for self, feelings about self, being treated as a person,* and *money.* Ratings of the single-item factors of *mental health* and *ability to make own decisions* decreased slightly from baseline to follow-up as being "very important" in determining quality of life perceptions of participants.

DISCUSSION

The significant changes in mean scores between baseline and follow-up on the quality of life domains of *importance of the environment, satisfaction with the environment, satisfaction with staff and care, satisfaction with activities and social relations, satisfaction with choice, satisfaction with the facility,* and *emotional well-being* suggest that the transition to FlexCare and an assisted living environment had a positive effect on program participants' perceptions of quality of life.

The change in environment and individualized care seemed to play a role in improving the emotional well-being of the participants. Assisted living participants reported significantly less anxiety and depression than they did when they resided in nursing homes. When not having to face depression, anxiety, or nervousness, participants were likely to take more interest or pleasure in the environment and activities with which they were surrounded. This, in turn, contributed to greater congruence with the environment. It was interesting to observe that while participants seemed to be less depressed/anxious after moving to the assisted living facilities, the family members/friends did not see them as having improved in this area. It may be important in further studies to see if this trend holds. Family members/friends may have projected some of their own feelings rather than accepting the adjustment of the participants.

In addition, participants residing in assisted living facilities reported a statistically significant higher level of satisfaction with their choices than they

TABLE 4. Importance of Single-Item Factors in Determining Quality of Life as Reported by Family Members/Friends: Nursing Home vs. Assisted Living Facility (N = 31)

Factors in Determining Quality of Life	Not at all Important				Slightly Important				Moderately Important				Very Important			
	Nursing Home		Assisted Living Facility		Nursing Home		Assisted Living Facility		Nursing Home		Assisted Living Facility		Nursing Home		Assisted Living Facility	
	#	%	#	%	#	%	#	%	#	%	#	%	#	%	#	%
Physical health	0	0	0	0	0	0	0	0	8	25.8	7	22.6	23	74.2	24	77.4
Mental health*	0	0	0	0	0	0	0	0	4	12.9	4	12.9	27	87.1	26	83.9
Family/friends	0	0	0	0	1	3.2	1	3.2	7	22.6	7	22.6	23	74.2	23	74.2
Ability to care for self*	0	0	1	3.2	3	9.7	2	6.5	13	41.9	9	29.0	15	48.4	18	58.1
Feelings about self	0	0	0	0	3	9.7	1	3.2	7	22.6	7	22.6	21	67.7	23	74.2
Being treated as a person	0	0	0	0	3	9.7	1	3.2	7	22.6	7	22.6	21	67.7	23	74.2
Ability to make own Decisions/choices	0	0	0	0	2	6.5	3	9.7	10	32.3	10	32.3	19	61.3	18	58.1
Money*	1	3.2	2	6.5	5	16.1	4	12.9	9	29.0	8	25.8	16	51.6	17	54.8

* 1 participant did not respond to this item at follow-up.

did when living in the nursing home setting. The questions in this domain measured participants'satisfaction with opportunities to make their own decisions concerning daily activities, care and assistance, and use of the telephone. It may be that the individualized care and the less-restrictive, home-like atmosphere of the assisted living setting influenced participants'responses to these questions. Maintaining a perceived sense of control and choice appeared to be a major factor in preventing depression and learned helplessness among residents in long-term care facilities.

It was interesting to note that the single-item factors were mostly rated higher at follow-up for participants, which indicated that the FlexCare case management approach coupled with the assisted living facility environment may have given participants a more positive outlook.

The finding that the domains of *importance of environment, importance of staff activities*, and *importance of choice* remained essentially level from baseline to follow-up for family members/friends was not surprising since the ratings scored at the top end of the domain scale at both times of measurement. In other words, family members/friends believed that environment, staff, activities, and choice were important in determining quality of life both at baseline and at the four-month follow-up. It may be that these ratings of "importance" wouldn't change from one setting to another and are just as important no matter where a person lives.

As with participants, family members/friends appeared to perceive improvement in both *domain* and *single-item* quality of life issues after the FlexCare participant changed housing arrangements. It appears that there is a strong trend for both participants and family members/friends to be more satisfied with the assisted living situation coupled with FlexCare case management. With this congruence between participants and family members/friends, it may be fair to conclude that quality of life did indeed improve with the group of 42 participants who moved from nursing homes to assisted living facilities under the support of the FlexCare program.

LIMITATIONS AND FUTURE RESEARCH

There were several limitations of this study. The sample size was relatively small but did represent approximately 25% of the total number of participants enrolled in the FlexCare program during the time of data collection. The program evaluation occurred concurrently with the development of the FlexCare demonstration project itself. So, although small, the sample may well be representative of FlexCare participants. Furthermore, only participants who chose to move to an assisted living facility once FlexCare services were in place were included in this study. No other less-restrictive, community-based alternative living arrangements were involved (e.g., family or own home, sheltered care, shared housing). This too, however, was reflective of the developmental stage of the FlexCare program during the data collection period.

Although the study sample was very homogenous, with the majority being women and White, it is consistent with the fact that women have a longer life expectancy than men and therefore, older women outnumber men within their peer group (Hooyman & Kiyak, 1999; Lassey & Lassey, 2001; U.S. Census Bureau, 2000). Also, the sample is reflective of the racial/ethnic composition of the community in which this study took place. However, the lack of racial/ethnic diversity may limit the ability to generalize findings of this study to the broader population of older adults.

Another limitation is that this study only included individuals residing in an urban or suburban area. The FlexCare program only operated in a metropolitan area at the time of the study. Therefore, findings of this study may not be applicable to older adults living in rural areas.

No measures of spiritual or cognitive well-being facets of quality of life were included in this study. It is likely that including measures of cognitive and spiritual well-being would prove to be substantial determinants of perceptions of quality of life. Including information regarding cognitive and spiritual well-being in a quality of life assessment tool has the potential to elicit a richer, more accurate measurement of older people's quality of life perceptions.

A final limitation of this study was that there was no way of considering any extraneous variables that may have affected changes in the perceptions of quality of life of participants from baseline to follow-up. For example, changes in health conditions or losses of loved ones were not recorded in any of the data collection. Only a change in the living arrangement of participants was known (i.e., moving from a nursing home at baseline to an assisted living facility at follow-up) and the extra support services that were implemented because of the individualized intervention services of the FlexCare program (e.g., case management, home health assistance, visiting nursing services, physical therapy). These potential extraneous factors may have skewed the perceptions of participants and/or family members/friends and contributed to the noted changes between baseline and follow-up.

In addition to compensating for the limitations of this study mentioned above, future research on quality of life of older adults might also include perspectives from primary care providers. Comparing perceptions of program satisfaction and quality of life of the older individuals, their family members/friends, as well as caregivers and providers would likely elicit more comprehensive assessments of the effectiveness and efficiency of a program and/or services received by participants and would give a more thorough indication of their quality of life (Abels, Gift, & Ory, 1994; Becker, 1995; Becker, 1998; Becker et al., 1993; Becker et al., 1995; Cairl et al., 1999; Diamond & Becker, 1999; Diaz & Mercier, 1996; Diaz et al., 1999; George, 1998; Peak & Sinclair, 2002; Rabiner et al., 1997; Rodgers, Herzog, & Andrews, 1988; Rubenstein, Moss, & Kleban, 2000; Sainfort, Becker, & Diamond, 1996).

Conducting quality of life studies using a longitudinal approach is another way to strengthen future research in this area. An outcome captured at one single point in time, in one setting is rarely a true measure of meaningful impact (Lamb, 2001). Changes in living arrangements and/or care and services provided to older individuals may result in a temporary "honeymoon" period or may elicit "grateful testimony" reflecting the participants' being glad to be out of the nursing home and in a new community-based environment with individualized care and support services (Baker & Intagliata, 1982). Having at least two follow-up time periods of measurement post baseline may eliminate any "honeymoon" effects or minimize any effects of "grateful testimonies" on perceptions of quality of life of older individuals.

Because of the subjective nature of quality of life measures, qualitative studies designed to ask more open-ended questions may help to build theory in this area, define and conceptualize quality of life more accurately, and help guide evaluations of quality of life of older adults. In addition, qualitative findings may support or substantiate findings of quantitative research such as those from this study.

Research involving larger sample sizes would strengthen quality of life studies. Findings would likely be more generalizable to the broader population of older adults. Also, conducting a study that includes a control group might be worthwhile. For example, it would be interesting to compare the perceptions of older individuals enrolled in the FlexCare program with those who are eligible but did not choose to receive program services. Are there any differences in quality of life perceptions between these two groups? Further studies may also consider quality of life perceptions of older people residing in other settings than nursing homes and assisted living facilities. For example, a future research question may ask, how do perceptions of quality of life of older people living in their own homes compare with those living in a sheltered care setting? Increasing the sample size, comparing other alternative settings, and using comparison and/or control groups may generate more definitive concepts of quality of life that may be used to measure perceptions of older adults in a more useful way. Having a better understanding of what constitutes quality of life for older adults will serve to assist service delivery systems to be more responsive to the interests of this population.

IMPLICATIONS AND CONCLUSIONS

This study found that the choice of housing arrangements relates to perceptions of quality of life of older adults. The concept of "quality of life" is a fluid concept and thus difficult to measure. Quality of life is relevant to a person's sense of being and how he/she fits into his/her own environment when trying to carry out daily activities. Daily activities themselves are always changing as the individual encounters the physical problems associated with the aging process. Feelings of self-worth and self-esteem may be the foundation upon which each individual defines his/her own–and very personalized–quality of life.

While acknowledging the difficulty of measuring quality of life issues, the data analysis of this study revealed that seven of the 14 participant domains and five of the 12 family member/friend domains improved significantly from when the FlexCare participant resided in a nursing home to when s/he resided in an assisted living facility. Participants rated themselves as being significantly less depressed. While this study is exploratory in nature and is limited to only four months, it demonstrates that quality of life issues can be addressed and that changes in these issues can be measured.

Viewing health and well-being from a holistic perspective rather than looking at only one facet of health and well-being, provides a means for improving individuals' lives through care plans, health-promotion activities, and community development. This holistic approach is consistent with social work practice theory and the environmental press framework. The findings of this study contradicted much of the literature which emphasizes the use of only one assessment model to ascertain perceptions of quality of life–the most dominant being health-related quality of life measures (Baxter & Shetterly, 1998; Bond, 1999; Cairl et al., 1999; Farquhar, 1994; Farquhar, 1995; Galambos, 1997; Livingston et al., 1998; Marinelli & Plummer, 2001; Noelker & Harel, 2001; Osberg et al., 1987; Raphael, Brown, Renwick, & Rootman, 1997; Steiner et al., 1996). Based on the results of this study that support the argument that multiple facets of life be more evenly considered in the measurement of quality of life, it is particularly important to incorporate environmental factors into quality of life measurements, especially a person's living arrangement.

Although quality of life is difficult to measure, it is important because a great many aspects of the lives of older adults are affected by service policy or programming changes (Kane, 2001; Kane & Kane, 2001; Raphael et al., 1997). Assessment within acceptable quality of life domains can serve as an indicator of needs and gaps in services. Identifying factors that enhance quality of life along with factors that reduce it, from multiple perspectives, within the application of the environmental press framework, can help social workers better address the needs of older adults. It may also guide program evaluation and, in effect, improve existing services. The findings of this study support the creation of innovative, more flexible approaches to providing long-term care and housing options for older adults, such as those provided by the FlexCare program, which solely utilizes Medicaid funds. By taking individual preferences and choices into consideration without limiting the available resources (e.g., Medicaid) to meet their needs, choices of care and support services can be made available that maximize quality of life for older people and foster their independence. Investigations such as this hold promise as our society struggles to provide care and housing alternatives for the increasing numbers of older adults.

As the demographic composition of the United States changes and the needs of older and/or disabled adults change, services will need to be modified in order to accommodate those needs in a way that optimizes societal and individual perspectives of quality of life.

The findings of this study are significant in that they support the use of Medicaid monies to allow nursing home-eligible, low-income older adults and/or individuals with a disability to have an array of long-term care and housing arrangements from which to choose. In addition, the participants utilizing the different long-term care settings have the advantage and support of individualized care through FlexCare case management. The choice of housing arrangements and the support of the FlexCare program seem to have improved the participants' perceptions of their quality of life.

REFERENCES

Abels, R. R., Gift, H. C., & Ory, M. C. (1994). *Aging and quality of life.* New York: Springer Publishing Company.

Arnold, S. B. (1991). The measurement of quality of life in the frail elderly. In J. E. Birren, D. E. Deutchman, J. E. Lubben, & J. Cichowlas-Rowe (Eds.), *The concept and measurement of quality of life in the frail elderly* (pp. 50-73). San Diego, CA: Academic Press, Inc.

Atchley, S. (1991). A time-ordered, systems approach to quality of assurance in long-term care. *The Journal of Applied Gerontology, 10* (1), 19-34.

Baker, F., & Intagliata, J. (1982). Quality of life in the evaluation of community support systems. *Evaluation Program Planning, 5*, 66-79.

Barusch, A. S. (1991). *Caring for the frail elderly.* New York and London: Garland Publishing.

Baxter, J., & Shetterly, S. M. (1998). Social network factors associated with perceived quality of life. *Journal of Aging & Health, 10*(3), 287-311.

Becker, M. (1995). Quality of life instruments for severe chronic mental illness: Implications for pharmacotherapy. *PharmocoEconomics, 7*(3), 229-237.

Becker, M. (1998). A U.S. Experience: Consumer responsive quality of life measurement. *Canadian Journal of Community Mental Health, 3*, 41-52.

Becker, M., Diamond, R., & Sainfort, F. (1993). A new patient focused index for measuring quality of life in persons with severe and persistent mental illness. *Quality of Life Research, 2*, 239-251.

Becker, M., Shaw, B., & Reib, L. (1995). *Quality of life assessment manual.* Madison: University of Wisconsin.

Bond, J. (1999). Quality of life for people with dementia: Approaches to the challenge of measurement. *Ageing and Society, 19*, 561-579.

Bradburn, N. (1969). *The structure of well-being.* Chicago: Aldine.

Braun, K. L., & Rose, C. L. (1989). Goals and characteristics of long-term care programs: An analytic model. *The Gerontologist, 29*(1), 51-58.

Brink, S. (1997). The greying of our communities worldwide. *Ageing International, Winter/Spring*, 13-31.

Brink, T., Yesavage, J., & Lum, O. (1982). Screening test for geriatric depression. *Clinical Gerontology, 1*, 37-43.

Brown, D. (1995). *Minimum data set version 2 reference manual.* Washington, DC: Eliot Press.

Bury, M., & Holme, A. (1990). Quality of life and social support in the very old. *Journal of Aging Studies, 4*(4), 345-357.

Cairl, R., Pfeiffer, E., & Keller, D. (1984). *Geriatric assessment testing and evaluation system.* Suncoast Gerontology Center, University of South Florida Medical School.

Cairl, R. E., Schonfeld, L., Becker, M., & Oakley, M. (1999). *The Florida quality of life and care (QLAC) assessment system project.* Report to the Florida Agency for Health Care Administration. Unpublished document.

Diamond, R., & Becker, M. (1999). The Wisconsin Quality of Life Index: A multidimensional model for measuring quality of life. *Journal of Clinical Psychology, 60(supplement 3)*, 29-31.

Diaz, P., & Mercier, C. (1996). An evaluation of the Wisconsin Quality of Life Questionnaires for clinical application and research in Canada. *Quality of Life Newsletter, 16*(2), 11-12.

Diaz, P., Mercier, C., Hachey, R., Caron, J., & Boyer, G. (1999). An evaluation of psychometric properties of the client's questionnaire of the Wisconsin Quality of Life Index-Canadian version (CaW-QLI). *Quality of Life Research, 8*, 509-514.

Eng, C., Pedulla, J., Eleazer, P., McCann, R., & Fox, N. (1997). Program of all-inclusive care for the elderly (PACE): An innovative model of integrated geriatric care and financing. *Journal of American Geriatric Society, 45*, 223-232.

Farquhar, M. (1994). Quality of life in older people. *Advances in Medical Sociology, 5*, 139-58.

Farquhar, M. (1995). Elderly people's definitions of quality of life. *Social Science and Medicine, 41*(10), 1439-1446.

Franks, J. S. (1996). *Residents in long-term care: A case-controlled study of individuals in nursing homes and assisted living in Washington state.* Unpublished doctoral dissertation, University of Washington, Seattle.

Galambos, C. M. (1997). Quality of life for the elder: A reality or an illusion? *Journal of Gerontological Social Work, 27*(3), 27-44.

George, L. K. (1998). Dignity and quality of life in old age. *Journal of Gerontological Social Work, 29*(2/3), 39-52.

Hooyman, N., & Kiyak, H. A. (1999). *Social gerontology: A multidisciplinary perspective.* Needham Heights, MA: Allyn & Bacon.

Hughes, S. L., & Guihan, M. (1990). Community-based long-term care: The experience of the living at home programs. *Journal of Gerontological Social Work, 15*(3/4), 103-129.

Kane, R. A. (2001). Long-term care and a good quality of life: Bringing them closer together. *The Gerontologist, 41*(3), 293-304.

Kane, R. L., & Kane, R. A. (2001). Emerging issues in chronic care. In R. H. Binstock & L. K. George (Eds.), *Handbook of aging and the social sciences (5th Edition).* San Diego: Academic Press.

Lamb, G. S. (2001). Assessing quality across the care continuum. In L. S. Noelker & Z. Harel (Eds.), *Linking quality of long-term care and quality of life.* New York, NY: Springer Publication Company.

Lassey, W. R., & Lassey, M. L. (2001). *Quality of life for older people: An international perspective.* Upper Saddle River, NJ: Prentice Hall.

Livingston, G., Watkin, V., Manela, M., Rosser, R., & Katona, C. (1998). Quality of life in older people. *Aging & Mental Health, 2*(1), 20-23.

Lucksinger, M. K. (1994). Community and the elderly. *Journal of Housing for the Elderly, 11*(1), 11-28.

Marinelli, R. D., & Plummer, O. K. (1999). Healthy aging: Beyond exercise. *Activities, Adaptation & Aging, 23*(4), 1-11.

McDowell, I., & Newell, C. (1987). *Measuring health: A guide to rating scales and questionnaires.* New York: Oxford University Press.

National Association of Social Workers. (1996). *Code of Ethics.* Washington, DC: Author.

Neugarten, B., Havighurst, R., & Tobin, S. (1961). The measurement of life satisfaction. *Journal of Gerontology, 16*, 134-143.

Noelker, L. S., & Harel, Z. (2001). Humanizing long-term care: Forging a link between quality of care and quality of life. In Noelker, L. S., & Harel, Z. (eds.), *Linking quality of long-term care and quality of life.* New York, NY: Springer Publication Company.

Osberg, J. S., McGinnis, G. E., DeJong, G., & Seward, M. L. (1987). Life satisfaction and quality of life among disabled elderly adults. *Journal of Gerontology, 42*(2), 228-230.

Ozawa, M. N. (1999). The economic well-being of elderly people and children in a changing society. *Social Work, 44*(1), 9-19.

Peak, T., & Sinclair, V. (2002). Using customer satisfaction surveys to improve quality of care in nursing homes. *Health & Social Work, 27*(1), 75-79.

Rabiner, D. J., Arcury, T. A., Howard, H. A., & Copeland, K. A. (1997). The perceived availability, quality, and cost of long-term care services in America. *Journal of Aging & Social Policy, 9*(3), 43-66.

Raphael, D., Brown, I., Renwick, R., & Rootman, I. (1997). Quality of life: What are the implications for health promotion? *American Journal of Health and Behavior, 21*(2), 118-128.

Rodgers, W. L., Herzog, A. R., & Andrews, F. M. (1988). Interviewing older adults: Validity of self-reports of satisfaction. *Psychology & Aging, 3*(3), 264-272.

Rosenberg, G., & Holden, G. (1997). The role of social work in improving quality of life in the community. *Social Work in Health Care, 25*(1/2), 9-22.

Rubenstein, R. L, Moss, M., & Kleban, M. H. (2000). *The many dimensions of aging.* New York, NY: Springer Publishing Company.

Sainfort, F., Becker, M., & Diamond, R. (1996). Judgements of quality of life of individuals with severe mental disorders: Client self-report versus provider perspectives. *American Journal of Psychiatry, 153*(4), 497-502.

Spitzer, R., Williams, J., Kroenke, K., Linzer, M., Verloin, G., Hahn, S., & Brody, D. (1995). *Prime-MD clinician evaluation guide.* New York: Pfizer, Inc.

SPSS, Inc. (2003). *Statistical Package for the Social Sciences, Version 11.5 software program.* Chicago: Author.

U.S. Census Bureau (2000). *2000 Census of population.* Retrieved March 23, 2002 from *http://quickfacts.census.gov/qfd/states/49/49011.html.*

Ware, J. E., & Sherbourne, C. (1992). The MOS 36 item short form health survey (SF-36). *Medical Care, 20*(6), 473-483.

Wright, S. (1999). Aging in the intermountain west: Demographic trends. *Intermountain Aging Review, 1*(1), 34-38.

doi:10.1300/J083v49n03_12

HISTORICAL PERSPECTIVES

Harriet Tubman's Last Work: The Harriet Tubman Home for Aged and Indigent Negroes

Sandra Edmonds Crewe, PhD, MSW

SUMMARY. This article focuses on the important contributions the venerable Harriet Tubman made to the field of housing for older persons and other populations at risk. It uses an historical approach to document the importance of early housing and self-help initiatives in the African American community. It embraces Harriet Tubman and other early housers for their good works and acknowledges them as contributors to the rich legacy of community social work practice and its sage principles of empowerment and self-help. The article presents a nexus between the

This paper is based on the paper *Harriet Tubman: Continuing Her Legacy as a Compassionate Houser for the African American Elderly*, presented at the Elmer Martin Memorial Lecture of the National Association of Black Social Workers in Jacksonville, Florida Adam's Mark Hotel. Jacksonville, FL (April 2003).

[Haworth co-indexing entry note]: "Harriet Tubman's Last Work: The Harriet Tubman Home for Aged and Indigent Negroes." Crewe, Sandra Edmonds. Co-published simultaneously in *Journal of Gerontological Social Work* (The Haworth Press, Inc.) Vol. 49, No. 3, 2007, pp. 229-244; and: *Housing for the Elderly: Policy and Practice Issues* (ed: Philip McCallion) The Haworth Press, Inc., 2007, pp. 229-244. Single or multiple copies of this article are available for a fee from The Haworth Document Delivery Service [1-800-HAWORTH, 9:00 a.m. - 5:00 p.m. (EST). E-mail address: docdelivery@haworthpress.com].

current housing status of older Blacks and the double jeopardy status imposed by historical discrimination. doi:10.1300/J083v49n03_13 *[Article copies available for a fee from The Haworth Document Delivery Service: 1-800-HAWORTH. E-mail address: <docdelivery@haworthpress.com> Website: <http://www.HaworthPress.com> © 2007 by The Haworth Press, Inc. All rights reserved.]*

KEYWORDS. African American elders, housing, historical research, double jeopardy

INTRODUCTION

In July 1896, at the first National Federation of Afro-American Women's conference in Washington, DC, Harriet Tubman used her celebrity status to talk on the theme of "More Homes for Our Aged" (Quarles, 1988, p. 50). Many social workers are aware of her acts of courage as a conductor of the Underground Railroad and a Civil War veteran, yet, much less is known about her service as a *caregiver* and *houser* for older persons (Martin & Martin, 1995). A *houser* is a person committed to raising the quality of life through improving availability of and access to shelter for low-income families (Oberlander & Newbrun, 1999). Remarkably, in her mid sixties, she developed a home for the aged in Auburn, New York. Social work and gerontological literature for the most part have omitted Harriet Tubman's role as a houser of the aged. While a few authors like Martin and Martin (1995, 2003) have mentioned her work, no publication has specifically heralded her contribution to the fields of gerontology, social work, and housing. According to Iris Carlton-Laney, an advocate for correcting history to include the accomplishments of African Americans:

> Accurate and cogently written social work history can be of great benefit to contemporary social work practitioners. It can help to connect present problems and future solutions with their historical antecedents. In addition to filling the gaps in our knowledge, history can also add dimensions of time to the practice of helping in the context of physical, socioeconomic, and cultural environments. (2001, p. i)

This article focuses on the important contributions the venerable Harriet Tubman made to the field of housing for older persons and other populations at risk. It uses an historical approach to present an overview of Harriet Tubman's life and documents the importance of early housing and self-help initiatives in the African American community. It presents a message of hope that is intended to encourage more social workers to become gerontological *housers* in the spirit of Harriet Tubman. It embraces Harriet Tubman and her collaborators and acknowledges their contributions to the rich legacy of community social work practice and its sage principles of empowerment and self-help. The article also addresses the continuing problem of double jeopardy, being both old and black, and its relationship to the lack of quality housing for African Americans. Additionally, the reader is made aware of other pioneering efforts in providing housing for African American elders. Finally, the author presents implications and recommendations for social work practice.

DOUBLE JEOPARDY HYPOTHESIS

Being Black and old in the United States has historically resulted in challenges for many who have been placed in "double jeopardy" because they face both the expected vicissitudes of aging with the added burden of racial discrimination. Being "black and old after a lifetime of racial discrimination" (Caliman, 1995, p. 1). The 1964 National Urban League publication, *Double Jeopardy–The Older Negro in America Today,* stated:

> Today's aged Negro is different from today's aged White because he is Negro ... and this alone should be enough basis for differential treatment. For he has, indeed, been placed in double jeopardy: first, by being Negro and second by being aged. Age merely compounded the hardships accrued to him as a result of being Negro. (p. i.)

The *Double Jeopardy* report publication along with a report for the Senate Aging Committee compiled by Dr. Inabel Lindsay, former Dean of the Howard University School of Social Work, emphasized the interrelationship between age and race. The report entitled *The Multiple Hazards of Age and Race: The Situation of Aged Blacks in the United States,* was presented at the 1971 National Conference on the Black Elderly where Dr. Lindsay outlined what had been presented at a special concerns session on aging Blacks at the 1971 White House Conference on Aging. Among the key recommendations were the creation of more housing for low and moderate income elderly, development of related social programs aimed at increasing the quality of life and the establishment of a National Caucus for the Black Aged in 1972 (Caliman, 1995).

Today there is continued evidence of double, triple, and quadruple jeopardy as gender and poverty are added as additional liabilities to the aging process (Crewe, 2003). The 2000 census provides evidence that neither the Emancipation Proclamation nor Civil Rights legislation have erased the disparities related to being born and aging in poverty. The 2000 census data report 2,787,427 non-Hispanic Blacks who are 65 and older (U.S. Bureau of Census, 2000). Of the nearly 35 million persons who are 65 or older, African Americans represent just over eight percent. Evidence of double jeopardy of the 65 and older Blacks can be seen in the census data that reveal that 44% of Black population as compared to 72% of Whites, have a high school degree or higher; 54% Blacks, as compared to 74% Whites, live with spouses; and 7% Blacks, compared to 2.7% Whites, live with non-relatives. Poverty rates are highest among minorities, especially Black women. The 1999 net worth of older Black households was $13,000 compared to $181,000 for older white households, a difference of $168,000. Additionally, the life expectancy at birth for Blacks continues to trail behind Whites by six years. Consistent with the 2000 census data, an Administration on Aging "Profile of Older Americans: 2003" shows that 23.8% of elderly African Americans were poor as compared with 8.3% elderly whites (U.S. Bureau of Census, 2003. These data clearly confirm the existence of double jeopardy and its adverse impact on housing options for poor elderly Blacks.

DOUBLE JEOPARDY IN HOUSING

The housing status of older Blacks is inextricably linked to earlier discrimination patterns in employment, housing, and access to social programs and benefits such as social security. Civil Rights legislation has been unable to level the playing field for persons who were denied basic rights over half their adult lives. As one of the fastest growing cohorts, older persons in the African American community came of age during times of segregation. This experience has defined their economic and social outcomes. Having overcome great obstacles, many have a great spirit of resilience that is reflective of Harriet Tubman. Siegel (1999) reminds us that Blacks who reached age 75 in 1998 were middle-aged when the Civil Rights movement occurred and reached retirement during the economically troubled years of the late 1970s and early 1980s. The earlier inequalities suffered by Blacks compounds their fragile economic state. Consequently, compared to Whites, nearly three times the proportion of older African Americans live below the poverty line (Hooyman & Kiyak, 2002) and are forced to rely more heavily on family and informal supports for their well-being.

The housing status of older Black Americans is uniquely different from their White counterparts, with differences likely reflecting the different value systems toward in-home versus institutional care and the limited availability and affordability of the range of housing options. Ozawa and Tseng (2000) report that even when other variables were held constant, the net worth of Black people was 90% less than the net worth of White people. This enormous difference in net worth translates directly to housing opportunities in old age. The National Association of Social Workers (NASW) acknowledges the inadequacy of today's housing options for persons who are poor and as such advocates for a national housing policy that "views housing as a social utility and a basic human need for all groups" (NASW, 2003, p. 197). The U.S. Department of Housing and Urban Development (HUD) also reports a small but growing number of elderly among the homeless (HUD, 2004). The federal housing programs established in 1959 for older persons continue to serve millions of families (Gelfand, 1999; Kart & Kinney, 2001), but new initiatives are needed to address the continuum of needs, range of incomes, and desire for choices that are culturally sensitive and maximize one's quality of life. Poor families as they age should be able to remain in the community and be supported by a range of housing and support programs.

The existence of continued disparities in housing choices requires a renewed commitment to developing programs and policies that focus on the needs of African Americans and other older persons who find themselves at the end of their lives with limited housing choices. More importantly, it requires greater involvement of African American social workers in collaboration with others committed to quality and affordable housing.

There is a rich legacy of self-help in the African American community and there is no time more important than today to rekindle the earlier efforts of pioneers in housing such as Harriet Tubman. The following profile of her life, and more particularly her housing legacy, provide shoulders to stand on as social workers face today's realities of shrinking support for housing and social service programs such as HOPE VI, Community Development Block Grant (CDBG), Community Services Block Grant (CSBG) and other federal programs that provided need housing for older persons.

HARRIET TUBMAN–EARLY YEARS

Harriet Tubman was born Araminta Ross around 1820 in Dorchester County, Maryland (Benge & Benge, 2002; Clinton, 2004a; Humez, 2003; Janney, 1999; Petry, 1955). Called Minty for short, she was born to parents Benjamin Ross and Harriet Green known as *Old Rit* in a windowless cabin on the Brodas plantation on Maryland's eastern shore. At the age of 13, her childhood ended abruptly when an overseer fractured her skull when she refused to restrain a fellow slave who was being beaten. This injury resulted in her having a disability that biographers described as somnolence, or a lethargic sleep that would come and go without warning (Benge & Benge, 2002; Clinton, 2004a;

Humez, 2003; Janney, 1999; Petry, 1955). This was a disability that she carried into older age.

In 1844, she married John Tubman, a free man. She yearned for freedom and despite her inability to get her husband to join her in her journey north, Harriet Tubman escaped alone in 1849 and sought asylum in Philadelphia; thus ending 28 years of enslavement. She was aided by her faith and reportedly the collaboration of a White lady whom she repaid with a prized bed quilt that she had pieced together (Humez, 2003; Clinton, 2004a). An October 3, 1849 notice described her as "MINTY, aged 27 years, is a chestnut color, fine looking, and bout 5 feet high" (Clinton, 2004a, p. 34). Her escape to freedom is heralded as the beginning of a movement, in which she became a navigator for hundreds of individuals and many others who sought freedom and a better quality of life.

THE UNDERGROUND RAILROAD YEARS

Once freed, as was customary for many formerly enslaved persons, Araminta assumed a new name, taking the name of her mother, Harriet. She was strongly committed to family and after escaping to freedom, she recognized the hollowness of freedom absent family members to share it with her (Martin & Martin, 1995). As a result she committed herself to reuniting family members separated by the institution of slavery. During the early 1850s, Harriet Tubman began her work with the Underground Railroad, reportedly rescuing over 300 enslaved people (Benge & Benge, 2002; Clinton, 2004a; Humez, 2003; Janney, 1999; Petry, 1955). Family members were among the enslaved persons that she navigated to freedom using the "North Star" (Bradford, 1886, p. 17; Clinton, 2004, p. 34; and Humez, 2003, p. 218). This illiterate yet visionary champion of freedom used her faith and wit to work toward an end to the cruel institution of slavery.

Although Canada was her base during the Underground Railroad years, she later resettled in Auburn, New York, a major station of the Underground Railroad. In 1857, William Seward, Governor of New York and avid supporter of Tubman, presented her with the deed to a house in Auburn. To avoid any appearance of charity, she asked to make a small regular series of payments. She later paid off the mortgage from the $1,400 in proceeds from the sale of a book about her life "Scenes in the Life of Harriet Tubman" written by Sarah Bradford in 1869.

One of Harriet Tubman's most remarkable accomplishments was escorting her aged parents to freedom. Ironically, some historians recorded this as one of the low points in her profile of courage–the uprooting of elders. While no justification is needed for wanting her aging parents to experience freedom, there was a compelling circumstance for her decision to rescue her parents. Shortly after moving to her home in Auburn, Harriet Tubman was notified that her father, now in his seventies, was awaiting trial for helping a fellow enslaved African. In response, in 1857, at the age of 37, Harriet engineered the escape of her mother and father who were both elderly. This escape is described as "a model of simplicity–and extraordinary daring" (Taylor, 1991, p. 69), with Tubman boldly driving her aged parents out of the south in the openness of a horse-drawn wagon. As cited by Taylor (p. 69), Biographer Earl Conrad (1943) stated:

> Harriet's abduction of her parents was an event in Underground annals. It was significant, not only because rarely did aged folks take to the Road, but also because Harriet carried them off with audaciousness and an aplomb that represented complete mastery of the Railroad and perfect scorn of the white patrol. Her performance was that, at once, of the accomplished artist and the daring revolutionary. (p. 69)

As noted, there were those who felt that Harriet Tubman was cruel and wicked for uprooting her parents. In the 1860 book, *Pictures of Slavery and Freedom*, John Bell Robinson characterized the rescue of her parents as:

> A diabolical act of wickedness and cruelty ... the bringing away from ease and comfortable homes two old slaves over seventy years of age ... as cruel an act as ever performed by a child towards parents. To help elderly people to be free was in his words ... a thousand times worse than to sell young ones away. (Taylor, 1991, p. 70)

There are many other accounts of older enslaved persons attempting to and succeeding in escaping to freedom (Ruiz, 2001). This contradicts the beliefs that older persons resigned themselves to their enslaved plight. Without freedom, for many there could be no comfort in old age. Like Harriet Tubman's parents, freedom never left the minds of many older Blacks who were forced to live and die as enslaved persons. The rescue of her parents is perhaps the beginning of the formal documentation of Harriet Tubman's commitment to housing for older persons. She moved her parents to her home in Auburn where she cared for them for nearly 30 years. Both her mother and father lived to be centenarians.

In addition to caring for her older parents, Harriet Tubman took in others who found themselves in need of shelter and care. Individuals with nowhere else to turn always inhabited her home. In her biography, it was recorded that she wanted her last work to be devoted to caring for those for whom she had already risked so much (Janney, 1999).

CIVIL WAR YEARS

During the Civil War, Harriet Tubman reportedly served as a spy and nurse for the Union Army (Benge & Benge, 2002; Clinton, 2004a; Humez, 2003; Janney, 1999; Petry, 1955). Prior to taking on assignments, she made arrangements for the care of her elderly parents. Her skills as a conductor of the Underground Railroad proved to be important in scouting out enemy positions. While the literature is clear about her active involvement in the Civil War, it is less clear about the details of her service. The "informality" of her military role in part resulted in the reliance on letters and word of mouth accounts of her service (Humez, 2003). Despite the lack of formal records, there is credible evidence that Harriet Tubman contributed her services in many ways to the Union Army. The official report which appeared in the 1874 *Congressional Record* described her service as follows:

> The whole history of the case establishes conclusively the fact that her services in the various capacities of nurse, scout, and spy were of great service and value to the Government, for which no compensation was paid beside the support which was furnished ... Your committee are of the opinion that she should be paid for these services and to that end report back to accompanying bill as a substitute for H.R. 2711, appropriating the sum of $2,000 for services rendered by her to the Union Army as scout, nurse, and spy, and recommend its passage. (Clinton, 2004a, p. 202)

During the Civil War, she assisted formerly enslaved persons to adapt to a new life of working for wages. For example, she used her own money to erect a wash-house and she personally spent time teaching freed women to do washing to avoid dependency on governmental aid (Humez, 2003). Yet, her service went uncompensated. Martin and Martin (2002) state it took Congress more than 30 years before they finally awarded Tubman a pension of $30.00 month. Not surprisingly, she used the pension to support her home for the aged.

Caregiver and Houser for Older Persons

In the autumn of 1865, Tubman returned to her Auburn home and continued to care for her aged parents at 180 South Street (Clinton, 2004b). Disabled from injuries, Harriet Tubman experienced difficulties providing for her needs and the most basic needs of elderly parents and other kinfolk, refugees, and boarders who became her dependents (Humez, 2003). The end of the war did not bring an end to her concern about the welfare of others. For the next half century she actively raised funds for schools, collected and distributed clothing, and

gave assistance to the sick and disabled (Quarles, 1988). In the preface of Sa-
rah Bradford's 1886 biography *Harriet, the Moses of Her People*, Tubman's
household was described as:

> Very likely to consist of several old black people bad with rheumatiz,
> some forlorn wandering woman, and a couple of images of God cut in
> ebony. How she manages to feed and clothe herself and them, the Lord
> best knows. She has too much pride and too much faith to beg. (p. 6)

Another writer describes Harriet Tubman's caregiving this way:

> All these years her doors have been open to the needy ... The aged ... the
> babe deserted, the demented, the epileptic, the blind, the paralyzed, the
> consumptive all have found shelter and welcome. At no one time can I
> recall the little home to have sheltered less than six or eight wrecks of
> humanity entirely dependent on Harriet for their all. (Clinton, 2004a,
> p. 203)

In 1869, Harriet Tubman married Nelson Davis, a Civil War Veteran and one of
her boarders. In her seventies and suffering from prolonged and frequent bouts
of somnolence, Tubman made another bold move (Janney, 1999). In 1886, over
30 years after escorting her parents to freedom, Harriet Tubman purchased two
houses at an auction on 25 acres of land across from her home in Auburn for
$1,450 (Clinton, 2004a; Clinton, 2004b; Janney, 1999). Tubman describes the
transaction:

> They were all white folks but me, there, and there I was like a blackberry
> in a pail of milk, but I hid down in a corner, and no one knew who was
> bidding. The man began down pretty low, and I kept going up by the fif-
> ties. At last I got up to fourteen hundred and fifty and the other stopped
> bidding, and the man said, "All done. Who is the buyer?" "Harriet
> Tubman," I shouted. (Conrad, 1943, p. 220)

Tubman obtained the money needed to purchase the land through a loan secured
by mortgaging the new land. Taylor (1991) states Harriet had her "usual supply
of determination and optimism" (p. 101). Her target audience was "anyone in
need." She wanted to provide a refuge for the young and the old, the sick and the
healthy, and the blind and the sighted. Tubman wanted to make meaningful the
promise of freedom by caring for those unable to care for themselves. She had
used her own home since the end of the war and found the needs of the residents
to be greater than her resources. She used self-help tactics and other means to
support those not able to care for themselves. For example, residents helped to

grow their own food and more able residents cared for the infirm, reflecting the strengths of the African American family (Hill, 1997). Within the institution of slavery, with their diminished ability to work in the fields, many older persons were abandoned to the good will of other enslaved persons (Schneider & Schneider, 2001). Unfortunately, some enslaved elders were left to fend for themselves and often experienced extreme hardship in old age. Others relied on the charity of their fellow enslaved persons. This reality, coupled with the tradition of mutual aid, is likely to have influenced Harriet Tubman's vision of a home for the aged and the self-help culture it represented.

During the decade that Tubman managed the home, she lived next door and continued to support the home from her farming operations (Humez, 2003). By the mid 1890s she recognized that she would not be able to continue to support this enterprise and appealed to her church for help. As a part of her appeal for support, she offered to house ministers in exchange for their support although her primary focus was destitute elderly women (Humez, 2003). Humez also reported that Tubman explored turning the home over to the National Association of Colored Women (NACW) because of her priority placed on serving destitute elderly women although the offer was not accepted because the property was not free of debt. Tubman also continued to receive support from her white antislavery supporters. This sometimes caused friction with the AME Zion clergy (Clinton, 2004a; Petry, 1955) who advocated strongly for self-help actions within the Black community.

In 1896, Tubman reached agreement with the church deeding the land and her home to the Thompson Memorial African Methodist Episcopal Zion Church in 1903. The agreement stipulated that she would have a lifetime deed and the place would be maintained as a home for indigent and aged colored people (Clinton, 2004a). One of the buildings on the ground was called John Brown Hall to honor the donor's wishes, however, the AME Zion church called the project the Harriet Tubman Home. In 1908, the home opened and it housed 12-15 persons of all ages and conditions. This joint venture with the AME church made her dream a reality. Yet, there were problems. Harriet Tubman objected strenuously to the home imposing an admissions fee of $100.00. She had never asked for any funds from those in distress and felt it was unconscionable for the church to do so. She simply did not believe that it was right to take care of the destitute and sick by requiring them to turn over money they didn't have. The home administrators were equally forceful in their belief that the home could not survive or thrive as a free home. Tubman reportedly said to a reporter:

> When I gave the home over to Zion Church, what do you suppose they did? Why they made a rule that nobody should come in without a hundred

dollars. Now I wanted to make a rule that nobody could come in unless they had no money. What's the need of a home if a person who wants to get in has to have money? (Petry, 1955, p. 241)

Despite her objections, AME Zion adopted a funding plan which de-emphasized contributions and instead put in place a $150.00 fee that gave lifetime privileges (Humez, 2003). Additionally, annual collections were taken for the maintenance fund ($200) of the home.

Another area of discord between Tubman and the church was who should be on the board of directors. While she felt that the board should be interracial to leverage funds from the broader community, other board members felt that it was important to depend only on the Black community to support the home (Janney, 1999). Tubman did not doubt the African American community's desire to help, but she felt that they lacked the financial resources. She was outnumbered by board members who believed in a model of self-help emanating from within the African American community. This decision reflects the composition of trustees who were all African Americans and primarily ministers. Tubman was the only female on the board (Humez, 2003).

The five-bedroom home was dedicated in 1908. Coping with her own poverty and advanced age and frailty, Tubman moved into the home in 1911 and stayed until her death in 1913. During her last years she was aided by the Empire State Federation of Colored Womens Clubs. They organized a linen shower and voted to send $25.00 a month to further her comfort for the remainder of her life (Quarles, 1988). This group also paid for her funeral and the marble headstone that proclaimed her contribution to society. Tubman was buried with military honors and received widespread acknowledgements from both Blacks and Whites for her good works and compassion. Figure 1 shows hallmarks of her remarkable life.

The rebuilt Tubman home stands today as a national historic landmark preserving the humanitarian vision of its founder (Harriet Tubman Home for the Aged, 1998). The Harriet Tubman Home was designated as one of "America's Treasures" by then First Lady Hillary Clinton (Tubman's Home, 1999).

Other Early Examples of Self-Help Housing

Although the Harriet Tubman Home for Aged and Indigent Negroes serves as a beacon, the Tubman Home was not the first facility of its type for older African Americans. Philadelphia's Home for the Aged and Infirm Colored Persons (Stephen Smith Home) was opened in 1864 (Sabbath, 2001). Developed by Stephen Smith, a wealthy African American lumber merchant, through collaboration with various social services organizations, the Home served

FIGURE 1. Harriet Tubman Time Line

1820- Born in Dorchester, Maryland (approximate birth date)

1844- Married John Tubman

1849- Escaped from slavery in Dorcester, MD to Philadelphia, PA

1850- Started as conductor for Underground Railroad

1857- Purchased home in Auburn, New York (six acres) to care for her aged parents

1857- Planned and effected her parents escape from slavery

1863- Civil War Service as a nurse, spy, scout, practical teacher

1865- Returned home after Civil War to care for parents

1867- John Tubman (first husband) died

1869- Married Nelson Davis, Disabled Civil War Veteran

1871- Benjamin Ross (Father Died)

1880- Addressed a Rochester Susan B. Anthony Suffragette convention

1886- Purchased 25 acres of land for home for aged

1890- Applied for Civil War Veteran's pension

1892- Nelson Davis (second husband) died

1896- Helped to found the National Association of Colored Women (NACW)

1897- Congress authorized small widow's pension for life

1900- Granted $20.00 per month widow's pension for wartime services

1903- Deeded the land and her home to Thompson Memorial AME Zion Church

1911- Moved to the Tubman Home to receive care

1913- Died in Auburn, New York, Harriet Tubman Home

2003- Posthumously awarded pension balance for military service (Sen. Hillary Clinton)

as a provider of training for African Americans in Philadelphia and played a critical role in the development of the emerging field of housing and care for the aged.

Although Philadelphia is noted as the city with the first home for elderly African Americans, the Lemington Home for the Aged in Pittsburgh, Pennsylvania purports to be the oldest continuously African American-sponsored, long-term care organization (Oldest African American Nursing Home, June 24, 2004). Mary Peck Bond, an African American female, established the Lemington Home in 1877 and incorporated it six years later in 1883. It has been in operation for 127 years.

Stoddard Baptist Home in Washington DC is another example of African American leadership in long-term community-based care (Stoddard Baptist, n.d.). Established in 1902, it started as a home for pastors and their spouses. This home has existed for over 100 years. Marie T. Stoddard, a widely known white philanthropist of the late nineteenth century, provided the seed money. The 1902 edifice was located in southeast Washington, DC and was designed to serve eight elderly residents. The home relocated to a larger location in 1915. Today, the Stoddard Baptist Home is a 164-bed facility, with a staff of 200. Gloria Ducker, MSW, its chief executive officer, reports that the home has an 18 million dollar budget that includes private pay, Medicaid funds, and continued support from the area churches in Washington, DC (Gloria Ducker, personal communication, March 15, 2005).

These are exemplars of community-based and long-term care initiatives started in the late 1800s and early 1900s for African Americans. This history is significant given that almshouses and poor farms were the primary assistance used by states to care for the white elderly in the Unites States in the 1900s. The almshouses and poor houses were "known for their dilapidated facilities and inadequate care" (Evolution of Nursing Home Care, 2004, p. 1) and served as deterrents to governmental reliance (Young, 1999). However, during the reconstruction period, the African American aged population was cared for primarily by families and facilities developed specifically for Blacks. The "Negro Women's Clubs" and the Black church were often in the forefront of developing specific programs for the Black Aged (Hanson, 2003; Hodges, 2001).

Practice and Policy Implications

These accounts of Harriet Tubman's life clearly show the passion and compassion that she had for the poor–and in particular the aged poor. She neither was comfortable resting in her celebrity status and past successes, nor did she have the expectation that it was somebody else's job to do. Instead, she set out to make a difference and accomplished her dream of establishing a home for older African Americans.

Today, many older African Americans continue to experience hardship and inequity in housing. They need to experience the passion and compassion exhibited by Harriet Tubman to make sure that their voices are heard and that new ventures are being developed to meet their growing needs. This tribute to Harriet Tubman is a reminder of what can be accomplished if social workers are strong in their commitment to advocate for the housing needs for the elderly.

With the growing diversity in this population, it is imperative that social policies be adopted that respect the diversity and rights of older persons. The Tubman legacy is incomplete without the recognition of her immense contribution to the field of social work and elderly housing. Her efforts to foster self-help and empowerment is worthy of inclusion in practice courses. She faced the multiple challenges of being poor, female, and uneducated. Her resilience and determination allowed her to achieve much in her lifetime despite these considerable obstacles and challenges. Drs. Elmer and Joanne Martin (2003) in their book *Spirituality and the Black Helping Tradition*, acknowledged the importance of Tubman's faith in work with elders. Harriet Tubman referred to the Tubman Home for Aged and Indigent Negroes as her "last work" from the Lord (Janney, 1999). Martin and Martin noted that she used her own inadequate pension buttressed by faith to provide for her home. Today, faith-based initiatives are being promoted and Tubman's experiences can be used to both promote and critically examine the use of faith-based housing initiatives for older Blacks.

Another looming question today faced by practitioners is *who do we serve?* When there are declining resources, practice often embraces decision-making that is influenced by society's definition of the worthy vs. unworthy poor. Often worthiness is translated as to ability to pay. This debate continues today and is couched in dialogue about the worthy versus unworthy poor or the belief that participant's contribution to their own services adds value to the resource. Many low income programs require a contribution from the recipient of services to demonstrate their commitment to self-help. An example is minimum rent in public and assisted housing where residents must contribute an agency established minimum rent (up to $50) toward their housing (Minimum Rent Rule, 2004). This seems to be a good faith deposit that distinguishes a "hand-up" from a "handout." Similarly the Quality Housing and Work Responsibility Act of 1998 (QHWRA) contained a 8-hour monthly community service and self-sufficiency requirement that institutionalizes "giving something back" (US HUD, 2003, p. 1). Tubman also struggled with this same ethical dilemma and today social work practitioners can use her story to more carefully examine the issue of rationing services.

There are many lessons to be learned from studying the Tubman Home. Perhaps the paramount lesson is that more social workers must become *housers* and focus as Harriet Tubman did, on the needs of older persons who continue to be placed at risk because of cumulative race-based disadvantages. This double jeopardy can and must be addressed through collaboration, self-help, and linking with new and long-term partners. In closing, on the occasion of the 1908 dedication ceremony of the Tubman Home, her remarks challenge today's generation of gerontological social workers to take up her cause and advocate for housing: "*I did not take up this work for my own benefit but for those of my race who need my help. The work is now well started and I know God will raise up others to take care of the future. All I ask is united effort, for 'united we stand: divided we fall'*" (Humez, 2003, p. 327).

REFERENCES

Administration of Aging. (2003). A profile of older Americans: 2003. Retrieved March 15, 2005 at *http://www.aoa.gov/prof/Statistics/profile/2003/10.asp.*

Benge, J., & Benge, G. (2002). *Harriet Tubman.* Lynwood, Washington: Emerald Books.

Bradford, S. (1886). *Harriet, the Moses of her people.* (reprint, Mineola, New York: Dover Publications, Inc., 2004).

Caliman, N. M. (1995). *The National Caucus and Center for the Black Aged: A history of the National Caucus and Center on Black Aged 1970-1995.* Washington, DC: Author.

Carlton-Laney, I. (2001). *African American leadership.* Washington, DC: NASW Press.

Clinton, C. (2004a). *Harriet Tubman.* New York: Little Brown and Company.

Clinton, C. (2004b). Slavery is war. In David Blight (Ed.). *Passages to freedom: The underground railroad in history* (pp. 195-209). Smithsonian: Washington, DC.

Conrad, E. (1943). *Harriet Tubman.* Washington, DC: Associated Press.

Crewe, S. E. (2003). Elderly African American grandparent caregivers: Eliminating double jeopardy in social policy. In T. Bent-Goodley (Ed.). *African American perspectives of social welfare policy* (pp. 35-54). New York: Haworth Press.

Evolution of Nursing Home Care in the United States. Retrieved 7/24/04 at *http://www.pbs.org/newshour/health/nursinghomes/timeline.html.*

Gelfand, D. E. (1999). *Aging network: Programs and services.* New York: Springer Publishing Company.

Hanson, J. A. (2003). *Mary McLeod Bethune & Black women's political activism.* Columbia, MO: University of Missouri Press.

Harriet Tubman Home for the Aged (March 30, 1998). Retrieved 3/11/05 at *http://www.cr.nps.gov/nr/travel/pwwwmh/ny13.htm.*

Hill, R. B. (1997). *The strengths of the Black family: Twenty-five years later.* Washington, DC: R & B Publishers.

Hodges, V. G. (2001). Historical development of African American child welfare services. In Iris Carlton-Laney (Ed). *African American leadership: An empowerment tradition in social welfare* (pp. 203-213). Washington, DC: NASW Press.

Hooyman, N. R., & Kiyak, H. A. (2002). *Social gerontology: A multidisciplinary perspective,* 6th ed., Boston: Allyn & Bacon.

Humez, J. M. (2003). *Harriet Tubman.* Madison, Wisconsin: University of Wisconsin Press.

Janney, R. P. (1999). *Harriet Tubman.* Minneapolis, Minn: Bethany Press.

Kart, C. S., & Kinney, J. M. (2001). *The realities of aging: An introduction to gerontology (6th ed.).* Boston: Allyn & Bacon.

Martin, E. P., & Martin, J. M. (1995). *Social work and the Black experience.* National Association of Social Workers (NASW): Washington, DC.

Martin, E. P., & Martin, J. M. (2003). *Spirituality and the Black helping tradition in social work.* Washington, DC: NASW Press.

Minimum Rent Rule, 24 CFR, Section 5.630 (2004).

National Association of Social Workers [NASW] (2003). *Social work speaks: NASW policy statements (2003-2006)*. Washington, DC: NASW Press.

Oberlander, H. P., & Newbrun, E. (1999). *Houser: Catherine Bauer*. Vancouver: UBC Press.

Ozawa, M. N., & Tseng, H. (2000). Difference in net worth between elderly black people and elderly white people. In S. M. Keigher, A. E. Fortune & S. L. Witkin (Eds.), *Aging and Social Work: The Changing Landscapes* (pp. 67-82). Washington, DC: NASW Press.

Petry, A. (1955). *Harriet Tubman: Conductor on the underground railroad*. New York: Harper-Collins Publishers.

Quarles, B. (1988). Harriet Tubman: Unlikely leadership. In L. Litwack & A. Meier (Eds). *Black leaders of the nineteenth century* (pp. 43-47). Chicago: University of Illinois Press.

Ruiz, D. (2001). Traditional helping roles of older African American women: The concept of self-help. In I. Carlton-Laney (Ed). *African American leadership: An empowerment tradition in social welfare* (pp. 215-228). Washington, DC: NASW Press.

Sabbath, T. F. (2001). African Americans and social work in Philadelphia, Pennsylvania, 1900-1930. In I. Carlton-Laney (Ed). *African American leadership: An empowerment tradition in social welfare* (pp. 17-33). Washington, DC: NASW Press.

Schneider, D., & Schneider, C. J. (2001). *An eyewitness history of slavery in America*. New York: Checkmark Books.

Siegel, J. S. (1999). Demographic introduction to racial/Hispanic elderly populations. In T. P. Miles (Ed.). *Full-color Aging: Facts, goals, and recommendation for America's diverse elders* (pp. 1-19). Washington, DC: The Gerontological Society of America.

Stoddard Baptist Nursing Home (n.d.). Stoddard history. Retrieved March 15, 2005 at *http://www.stoddardbaptisthome.com/history.htm*.

Taylor, M. (1991). Harriet Tubman. New York: Chelsea House Publishers.

Tubman's Home for Aged Aided the Poor. *The Post Standard* (February 1, 1999) Retrieved 5/28/2004 *http://web.lexis-nexis.com*.

U.S. Bureau of Census (2000). Census 2000 data on aging. Retrieved March 15, 2005 at *http://www.aoa.gov/prof/Statatistics/Census2000/minority-sumstats.asp*.

U.S. Bureau of Census (2003). A profile of older Americans: 2003. Retrieved June 20, 2005 at *http://www.aoa.gov/prof/Statatistics/profile/2003/profiles2003.asp*.

U.S. Department of Housing and Urban Development [HUD] (2003). Notice PIH 2003-17. Reinstatement of the community service and self-sufficiency requirement.

U.S. Department of Housing and Urban Development [HUD] (2004). Homelessness. Retrieved March 15, 2005 at *http://www.aoa.gov/prof/homelessness/homeless ness.asp*.

Young, H. P. (1999). *Country folks: The way we were back then in Halifax County, Virginia*. Lawrenceville, Va: Brunswick Publishing Company.

doi:10.1300/J083v49n03_13

Index

Page numbers followed by and *f* or *t* indicate figures or tables.

245